OFFENDING WOMEN

SOCIOLOGY OF LAW AND CRIME

Editors:
Maureen Cain, University of the West Indies
Carol Smart, University of Warwick

This new series presents the latest critical and international scholarship in sociology, legal theory, and criminology. Books in the series will integrate the sociology of law and the sociology of crime, extending beyond both disciplines to analyse the distribution of power. Realist, critical, and post-modern approaches will be central to the series, while the major substantive themes will be gender, class, and race as they affect and, in turn, are shaped by legal relations. Throughout, the series will present fresh theoretical interpretations based on the latest empirical research. Books for early publication in the series deal with such controversial issues as child custody, criminal and penal policy, and alternative legal theory.

Titles in this series include

CHILD CUSTODY AND THE POLITICS OF GENDER
Carol Smart and Selma Sevenhuijsen (eds)

FEMINISM AND THE POWER OF LAW
Carol Smart

OFFENDING WOMEN

Female lawbreakers and the
criminal justice system

ANNE WORRALL

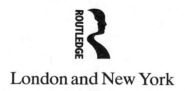

London and New York

11213817

First published 1990 by Routledge
11 New Fetter Lane, London EC4P 4EE

Simultaneously published in the USA and Canada by Routledge
29 West 35th Street, New York, NY 10001

Reprinted 1995, 1996

Routledge is an International Thomson Publishing company I(T)P

Typeset by Gilfillan Ltd, Mitcham, Surrey
Printed and bound in Great Britain by
Biddles Ltd, Guildford and King's Lynn

British Library Cataloguing in Publication Data
A catalogue record for this book is available from the British Library

Library of Congress Cataloguing in Publication Data
A catalogue record for this book is available from the Library of Congress

ISBN 0-415-03724-7 (hbk)
ISBN 0-415-03725-5 (pbk)

CONTENTS

SERIES EDITORS' PREFACE

It is no longer possible to introduce a book such as this with the assertion that there are virtually no studies of female law-breakers or of women and crime. Whether this is indicative of a desirable state of affairs is, however, debatable. There has grown up a veritable industry of texts on women and crime. Many are written from the stance of feminist empiricism, which seeks to increase the numbers of empirical studies of female offenders. Yet it remains questionable whether it is really adequate simply to render female offenders visible if the nature of that visibility is constructed through the parameters of a positivistic social science which seeks to control and remedy the women under investigation.

To a certain extent the study of women and crime seems to have found itself in a cul-de-sac. There is no feminist criminology; indeed it is arguable that this would be a contradiction in terms. Feminism seeks to deconstruct and liberate, while criminology seems inevitably to seek testable causes and feasible controls. This rejection of the 'coupling' of feminism with criminology may seem like mere pedantics, but there is a major theoretical crisis at the heart of much feminist work in the field of criminology.

This crisis is obscured and evaded by the empirical studies that simply seek to add to the quantum store of information. Others have avoided it by abandoning criminology for wider studies of regulation and analyses of other areas of law and policy. Yet others have addressed it indirectly by giving space to the expression of the subjectivity/ies of women law-breakers. This has allowed room for other kinds of knowledge to be disseminated. Perhaps most fruitful in recent years has been the study of women's imprisonment, in which we can clearly see a rejection of the pathologizing consequences of positivistic and liberal approaches. Studies of women's imprisonment have embraced a more robust theoretical perspective that avoids collusion with regulatory discourses.

This still leaves the problem of 'women and crime'. Should we ignore it and direct our gaze elsewhere, or should we seek to tackle the political and epistemological problem at the heart of the criminological project? Anne Worrall does the latter in the text that follows. Yet she does so without setting up 'women and crime' as her focus. Instead she concentrates on the formulation of knowledge about the woman who offends and how she resists the constructions that are imposed upon her. So Worrall does not concern herself with the unanswerable and futile question of why do women commit crimes, rather she looks at what passes for knowledge about such women. This knowledge she identifies as part of the regulation of these women, it is also part of their silencing. Women who offend are silenced, they become muted and unable to provide their own accounts of their subjectivity. The experts always already know these women and, through this knowledge, seek to manage them. Basing her work on interviews with the 'experts' and on the cases of fifteen women, Worrall approaches the question of women and crime from a perspective that opens up possibilities for new ways of understanding. What is to be found here is an unfolding of the issues rather than an intellectual closure. The disqualification of offending women is documented in considerable detail and we are able to see the continuum between this process and other (non-legal) procedures, which seek to render women passive and invisible. Ultimately this analysis breaks down the intellectual barriers between analyses of women in general and of women who offend. Many studies have argued that there is such a continuum, but few have been able to provide the analytical tools necessary to make the links.

Offending Women is a major contribution to the field of the sociology of law and crime. It will be relevant to scholars, policy makers, and practitioners. Undoubtedly it will challenge many preconceived notions and, in so doing, will make many of us feel uncomfortable as our role in the construction of 'expert' knowledge, and hence the management of 'troublesome' women, is exposed and examined.

Maureen Cain
Carol Smart
April 1989

ACKNOWLEDGEMENTS

I am grateful to the University of Keele for the award of a Studentship which funded the first year (1982–3) of the research on which this book is based.

I should like to thank the following people for their assistance:

Mr R.W.Harris, Chief Probation Officer, Staffordshire Probation Service, for permission to interview probation officers in Staffordshire.

All the people who allowed themselves to be interviewed – especially the women about whom this book is written.

Paul Wilding and Anne Kerr, who gently but persistently kept me to task. My colleagues in the Department of Social Policy and Social Work at Manchester University for their support and encouragement.

Andrew Worrall for his patience and understanding and Jennifer Worrall for helping me to keep a sense of perspective.

Pat Carlen, for whose invaluable help and encouragement over so many years this brief acknowledgement is wholly inadequate.

Finally, I dedicate this book to the memory of my mother, who experienced both the joy and the suffering that comes from struggling to defy description.

INTRODUCTION

Kathy, aged 20, is a good daughter and a normal young woman. She stabs her sister to death. The psychiatrist says she may suffer from epilepsy and if she's placed on probation he'll look into it. The judge calls it a tragic case – for Kathy. She is placed on probation for two years but the psychiatrist never asks to see her again. Ivy, aged 58, is charged with stealing a jar of coffee. She pleads 'not guilty'. She says she had just come out of psychiatric hospital and was still confused. She gives a very lucid account of herself – and is found guilty. She is placed on probation for three years, with a condition that she sees a psychiatrist regularly – which she does. Gwen, aged 38, put a brick through the window of her own council house. She is frustrated that she cannot get access to her daughter who is in Care. She is remanded in custody for psychiatric reports but a probation officer finds a hospital bed, where Gwen eventually remains for three months as a condition of a probation order.

Women like Kathy, Ivy, and Gwen are variously described as inadequate, demanding, manipulative, aggressive. While some might see them as 'feminist' clients (Wilson 1977), challenging the state's definitions of them and seeking to take control of their own lives, others may be left with the uneasy feeling that their behaviour exemplifies the 'defences of the weak' (Mathiesen 1972) – mere shadow-boxing by the powerless. Probation officers, social workers, solicitors, psychiatrists, and magistrates are all, from time to time, exercised by the demands to define these women who appear to defy description. Those demands emanate not only from the occupational ideologies within which such personnel consider themselves accountable, but also from the

1

ideologies within which the women see themselves as having been constituted. Indeed, it is often *their* apparent inability to define themselves outside the needs, demands, and definitions of other people that creates the greatest problems for those seeking to offer help. Such offers are frequently frustrated because the women appear to lurch constantly between two states of consciousness – a sense of obligation to fulfil the needs of husbands, cohabitees, mothers, children, neighbours – and a sense of outrage (at time suppressed into depression) that their own needs are not being met. And in the eyes of the agencies required to define them they more often than not appear to be *nondescript*.[1]

Such observations require explanation but those most commonly proffered are inadequate to account for both the specific plight of such women *and* the extent to which their experiences cast light on the experiences of other, non-criminal women. It may be true that women like Kathy, Ivy, and Gwen share with all women the absence of 'the right or the requirement to be full-fledged representatives of the culture' (Miller 1976: 76). But they also have a very particular experience which makes them different from other women. At some stage in their careers, they have broken the law and have been found out, thus immediately acquiring a statistically élite status and exposing themselves to the gaze of those whose interweaving official wisdoms – both expert and common-sensical – inform the criminal justice system. But that gaze, which traps Kathy, Ivy, and Gwen in the interstices of legal, psychiatric, and common-sense 'knowledge', leaves them ill-defined and unexplained. They are assessed, judged, treated, punished – not because they are understood, but because they are not.

Traditional theories of female crime have all been fundamentally positivistic in their nature. They have premised that it is possible to distinguish female law-breakers from non-law-breakers by characteristics other than their acts of law-breaking. These characteristics have been seen to reside within the individual physiology and psychology of generalized woman and/or specific women. While there may be some debate about whether such qualities are innate or socially determined, they are nevertheless presented as inherent, in the sense that they exist as more or less permanent, unified attributes. Consequently, these 'essential' qualities are viewed as widespread, if not actually universal, within the category 'female law-breaker' and can be

2

analysed ahistorically and without reference to any structural features of particular societies and cultures. In other words, the observed category, 'women who break the law', is assumed to correspond with an abstract category, part of a pre-existing universe of phenomena, about which 'knowledge' can be discovered through the classification of symptoms, the diagnosis of a syndrome, and the search for an aetiology.

In contrast, structural analyses of female crime have been forced to overlook the plight of the individual offender and have thus ultimately proved unhelpful to those for whom she is an inescapable reality. Valuable insights into the poverty and oppression which correlate with much female crime have been confounded by assertions that liberation from traditional social constraints will inevitably result in more crimes of affluence and violence among women. Such apparent incompatibilities have ironic consequences. Arguing for equality of exposure to public attention, equality of opportunity to commit crime, and equality of treatment by the criminal justice system at an individual level is not an obvious route to improving the lot of women. The advantages of discrimination in this arena for some women cannot be denied.

Instead, such analyses must draw attention away from individual offenders and concentrate on the social structure which produces 'specific systems, such as imperialism, racism, capitalism, and sexism, because they promote inherently repressive relationships and social injury' (Klein and Kress 1976: 36). The very definition of crime changes from that of individual law-breaking to that of anything which violates basic 'human rights to self-determination, dignity, food and shelter, and freedom from exploitation' (Klein and Kress 1976: 36). Justice becomes a political rather than a legal concept, and the traditional distinctions between offenders and victims are questioned.

Where does this leave women like Kathy, Ivy, and Gwen? How can one account for their experiences without reducing them, on the one hand, to individual pathology or, on the other, to the always and already known consequences of capitalism and patriarchy? Is there a way of moving from observation to explanation without falling into such empiricist or reductionist traps? Is it possible to extrapolate from an abundance of common-sense and professional observations about these troublesome women:

3

– the rules by which differential diagnoses and judgements are made;

– the material conditions of existence within which those rules acquire meaning; and

– the material consequences of those rules for the women who are constructed as the objects of various, often contradictory claims to knowledge?

And, having done that, is it possible to relate any of those discoveries to the experiences of other women?

This is a book about women who do not fit the stereotypes. It is about a particular group of women but it is also about all women. It is about the ways in which magistrates, solicitors, psychiatrists, and probation officers try to control a small but disproportionately demanding group of female law-breakers who do not fit into the two traditional stereotypical categories of 'the menopausal shoplifter' or 'the sophisticated criminal' (Worrall 1981: 92). And it is about the ways in which those women sometimes elude control. But the conditions and processes that overdetermine the fate of this group of deviant women are intrinsically no different from those within which 'conventional' women are also controlled. So the aim of this book is not to explain why some women commit crimes and why most do not. Nor is its task to establish 'the facts' that might account for the homogeneity of a particular group of female law-breakers. Rather, it is to examine the ways in which the authorization of professionals and experts to define certain women as being the type of woman who requires treatment, management, control, or punishment serves to perpetuate the oppression of all women. Similarly, by examining the ways in which certain women subtly resist such definitions, challenging and undermining their authority, the possibility is kept open of developing new understandings of the experiences of all women.

Reflects operation of agencies

way in which FO ~~act~~ tackel reflects all women.

not positivism (causes)

Chapter One

THEORIZING WOMEN'S EXPERIENCES

> Discourse analysis has displaced epistemology.
>
> (Burton and Carlen 1979: 15)

This book has two central concerns:

1) Under what conditions do certain people claim to possess knowledge about female law-breakers?

2) What is the process whereby such claims are translated into practices which have particular consequences for female law-breakers?

In order to ask these questions, it is necessary to adopt a methodology which avoids the pitfalls of conventional epistemology. Epistemology is concerned with how we discover truth. It struggles with distinctions between the natural and the social world, between causes and reasons. It asks whether knowledge is obtained by observing behaviour or understanding action, by accretion or by rational thought. It asks whether it is indeed possible for humans to study themselves at all or to have a full and absolute knowledge of themselves. In sum, it is concerned with the demarcation of science from non-science (of truth from falsehood), the relationship between theory and observation, and the conundrum of a knowing subject producing objective knowledge.

As opposed to dealing with questions of truth, however, this study struggles with the relationship between those who claim to know the 'truth' and those about whom they claim to know it. It searches for a method of analysis which reaches beyond what is said to be, to an understanding of what informs a particular claim to know. Its search is for the underlying structures whence emanate the rules that authorize such claims 'to know'. Its aim is to unhitch itself from the collusive search for properties, essences, and unities. Instead it asks, 'Why is there a need for agents of social control to reconstruct those they seek to control as though they were possessed of essential qualities?'

Starting from the premise that no human action is intrinsically meaningful and that no human being is endowed with pre-given properties or essences which transcend the social system and determine her or his lived experience, it is possible to challenge those idealist forms of knowledge which depend on notions of 'human nature'. But the rejection of positivistic explanations of human behaviour does not immediately lead away from the traditions of epistemology. Reacting against notions of truth as unchanging and monolithic, the notion of truth as a pluralistic realism is attractive. Truth may be a matter of perspective (Plummer 1979; Rock 1973). It may reside in neither subject nor object but in their interaction. Knowledge may not be the product of a priori reasoning nor may it inhere in the nature of the phenomena themselves. Knowledge may be:

– dialectic, for it is contradictory and uncertain;
– indeterminate, for it is dependent on changing conditions and contexts;
– pluralistic, for it is scattered among the minds of those who ask the questions;
– exploratory, for it cannot be reduced to axioms but is a mosaic built up through exploration.

Knowledge may never be total – it is better described as a process of knowing. Central to this knowing process is the 'knowing subject' – the 'self' that interacts with 'society' (Mead 1934). But the emergence of the self is a complex process, in which the acquisition of language is crucial. Through this process of maturing, it is argued, the individual comes to have a sense of herself as a 'single consistent coherent and organised personality' (Mead 1934: 269) with the power to anticipate, respond to, and influence her social environment.

But the women with whom this study is concerned most certainly did not experience themselves in this holistic and ordered way. On the contrary, they experienced internal conflict and a sense of self which was contradictory, inconsistent, and incoherent. Within this model of understanding, such experiences can only be described as pathological. Such an analysis reduces the problem of interaction to problems of consciousness. Consequently, their resolution lies in the raising of the social consciousness of individuals through increased knowledge of the complexity of human interaction and its consequences. Such an analysis is based on two fallacies: first, that knowledge alone and of itself leads to change and, second, that the 'self' is potentially as powerful as the forces which constitute 'society'. Underlying those two fallacies is a neglect of issues of power and structure, of the interrelation between consciousness and the material world in which it originates. The internalization of this consensus serves to pathologize internal conflict, rather than to view it as the product of social relations which are themselves products of inequalities of class, race, and gender.

The speaking subject does not have complete freedom to endow her words or her actions with meaning. She is not the centre of meaning or knowledge. Words and actions acquire socially determined meanings which exist independently of the intentions of the particular subjects who use those words or engage in those actions. It may be self-evident that there is nothing intrinsically polite about opening a door for a woman (Culler 1976: 92) but any intention on the part of a male subject to ascribe politeness to his action would be futile in an environment where the act itself was assumed to be patronizing. To understand the complexity of meaning that underlies such a ritual, one would have to go beyond the meanings articulated by the individual actors to an understanding of the relationships between conventions arising from idealist notions of chivalry and those arising from materialist discourses about women's oppression. The question which then arises is the extent, if any, to which the speaking (or knowing) subject plays any active part in that process. The subject has been 'de-centred' but has she become totally powerless?

The relationship between knowledge and power is crucial to any attempt to theorize women's experiences. The desire to know is a desire for power but knowledge of itself does not give power. On the contrary, it is those who have power who are authorized 'to know' and whose 'knowledge' is afforded privilege. But the process whereby such claims to know are authorized is a complex one, for power is not simply something which is produced by a particular class in society, transmitted through monolithic institutions, conspiratorial laws, and single-purpose systems. Power inheres in all social relations. Its origins are local and immanent, and its circulation through the social body can be likened to the capillary circulation of blood through the physical body (Hewitt 1983). The key to power is not overt domination of one group by another, but the acceptance by all that there exists 'an ideal, continuous, smooth text that runs beneath the multiplicity of contradictions, and resolves them in the calm unity of coherent thought' (Foucault 1972: 155). In other words, power is achieved whenever paradox is simultaneously affirmed and denied – whenever its surface appearance is acknowledged but its underlying implications repressed. For example, the judge presiding over Kathy's trial readily admitted the apparent paradox of placing a murderess on probation, but denied the existence of any underlying contradiction. This was, after all, a 'tragic case'. In contrast, it might appear paradoxical that Gwen should be hospitalized for damaging her own property, but *beneath the surface* lies an essentially sick personality.

This process of reconstructing paradox as coherence, of rendering 'that which is absent present' (Cousins 1978: 70) is the fundamental project of discourse. The term is used here to embrace all aspects of a communication – not only its content, but its author (who says it?), its authority (on what grounds?), its audience (to whom?), its object (about whom?), its objective (in order to achieve what?). Discourse

> appears as an asset – finite, limited, desirable, useful – that has
> its own rules of appearance, but also its own conditions of
> appropriation and operation; an asset that consequently, from
> the moment of its existence (and not only in its 'practice
> applications'), poses the question of power; an asset that is, by
> nature, the object of a struggle, a political struggle.
>
> (Foucault 1972: 120)

Analysis of discourse involves the deconstruction of coherence to reveal the underlying paradox and expose the absence of that which has been represented as being present. For example, one way of ensuring the 'infinite continuity of discourse' (Foucault 1972:25) is to demarcate its boundaries by employing 'practices of exclusion' (Gordon 1977:15). Such practices might include the prohibition of certain topics on grounds of 'irrelevance', the disqualification of certain individuals from being authorized speakers, and the rejection of certain statements as illegitimate. Gwen's poverty is irrelevant to an assessment of her mental health; Ivy is disqualified from speaking about her own guilt or innocence; Kathy is not to be described as a murderess.

PROGRAMMES, TECHNOLOGIES, STRATEGIES – AND RESISTANCE

What then is the relationship between discourse and practice? What are the mechanisms whereby, in the face of a fragmented and contradictory reality, claims to know can be successfully translated into effective unified knowledge with over-determined consequences?

First, that fragmented and contradictory reality has to be reconstructed as a field of recognizable (that is, unified and ideologically congruent) objects, in which it is possible to intervene on the basis of a priori existing knowledge. The observable phenomenon of women breaking the law has to be programmed as women *who break* the law, and about whom knowledge already exists – has always existed, waiting to be laid claim to. And that knowledge already contains within it (perversely hidden but ultimately reachable) its own inevitable consequences and 'correct' solutions.

Second, those programmes of power require a channel of conveyance. The technology of such conveyance is varied and disparate. It may consist of architectural institutions, like courtrooms, hospitals, schools, factories, or prisons; it may consist of practices such as the provision of welfare, the ascription of motives, or the practices of exclusion already discussed. Finally, it may consist of norms – technologies which have been internalized to the extent that they are no longer recognized as technologies at all. Self-regulation demonstrates the supreme success of a programme.

Third, and conceptually most elusive, programmes and technologies are dependent for their success on strategies of intervention. Strategy is not the coherent, logical, overall

9

planning of action (although it may be represented as such). Rather, it is an opportunistic and expedient means of exploiting the field of intervention. It is the means whereby the authority of programmes can be maintained (or denied) in spite of (and yet because of) their effects. Strategy is 'the outcome of a complex and fragmented process of struggle, within which the calculations of individuals and agencies play a crucial, but by no means controlling, part' (Garland 1985: 208). It is the process whereby individuals and agencies attempt to anticipate the effects of programmes and technologies and then utilize those effects to justify the continuance or cessation of such intervention. It is the means by which a programme 'caters in advance for the eventuality of its own failure' (Gordon 1979: 38).

At this point, however, there is a danger of losing sight of the speaking subject. What power, if any, does she have over this process? Programmes, technologies, and strategies give certain meaning – or signification – to the subject and her acts and foreclose on the possibility of alternative meanings. To the extent that this signifying code is accepted by the subject, then it holds and controls her. Nevertheless, the subject does have power – the power to 'infringe the code in the direction of allowing the subject to get pleasure from it, renew it or even endanger it' (Kristeva 1975: 52). The power of the subject is, therefore, the power of negativity and heterogeneity. It is the power to 'say "No" to the conditions of existence of existent knowledge' (Burton and Carlen 1979: 19); it is the power of resistance to and refusal of assumptions of homogeneity. By demonstrating the existence of heterogeneity and contradiction, the speaking subject is helping to keep open the space within which knowledge is produced.

But is the nondescript female law-breaker really a resister? Does she, in fact, defy description? Surely, to view her as such is merely to romanticize her plight? For the most part, female law-breakers appear markedly non-resistant. For the most part, they appear to be muted:

> The theory of mutedness ...does not require that the muted be actually silent. They may speak a great deal. The important issue is whether they are able to say all that they would wish to say, where and when they wish to say it. Must they, for instance, re-encode their thoughts to make them understood in the public domain? Are they able to think in ways which they

would have thought had they been responsible for generating the linguistic tools with which to shape their thoughts? If they devise their own code will they be understood?

(Ardener 1978: 21)

Members of muted groups, if they wish to communicate, must do so in terms of the dominant modes of expression. But dominance does not require the active domination of one group by another nor does it require any one individual's structural position in a society to be constant. It is dependent, rather, on a 'sub-group, or particular universe, of relevance at any one time' (Ardener 1978: 28), which produces:

– ideas about 'reality' and who is authorized to define it;
– the blunting of self-perceptions through the encouragement of 'trivial' concerns and small-scale pleasures;
– the exclusion of muted groups from 'public' space.

The subtlety of such dominance ensures that rebellion is confined to 'minor deviations' which 'can become charged with emotive force' for the participants but may exert little influence on the dominant group (Ardener 1978: 28-9).

Yet, on closer examination, such 'minor deviations' may have power after all. One of the victims in Foucault's compelling drama about a nineteenth-century French triple murderer, Pierre Rivière, is the protagonist's mother, Victoire. Unlike her son, her mode of resistance to intolerable conditions of existence is not florid homicidal psychosis but subtle elusiveness and a frustrating refusal to comply with contracts entered into. She

felt that any contract remained a trick, an institutionalized assault ...a frozen arrested, perpetual combat. She set herself up as an everlasting canceller of contracts, perpetually put them in doubt, and shifted their signs by setting them moving again – which is tantamount to repudiation and challenge.

(Foucault 1975: 181)

Female law-breakers may have their own programmes, technologies, and strategies, for 'the existence of those who seem not to rebel is a warren of minute, individual autonomous tactics and strategies which counter and inflect the visible facts of overall domination' (Gordon 1979: 43).

11

IMPLICATIONS FOR METHODOLOGY

The adoption of this particular mode of theorizing women's experiences calls for a method of research which rejects notions of generalization through probability in favour of generalization through theoretical production. I have not sought to argue that I have found sufficient examples of the coexistence or correlation of two or more characteristics in my sample to justify asserting their coexistence or correlation in a wider population. I have not, for example, argued that, because the majority of the magistrates in this sample claimed to have little experience of dealing with female defendants, it is therefore probable that most magistrates would make a similar claim. I have argued instead that such claims illustrate the theoretical construct of 'self-disqualification' – a construct which I believe capable of offering some insight into the attitudes and practices of magistrates. I have then attempted to identify the specific ideological and material conditions necessary for the production and reproduction of such a construct.

The interviews on which this book is based constitute a case study. The term is used here to mean a detailed examination of material (in this instance, statements about attitudes and practices relating to a particular group of female law-breakers) which I believe demonstrates the operation of a general theoretical principle (namely, the power of discourse). The selection of interviewees was not random (for more details, refer to the appendix on 'Researching Women') nor is it claimed that those selected were necessarily representative of the wider population of their profession or status. They were chosen in the expectation not that their statements would be typical but that they would provide compelling illustrations of (or challenges to) my theoretical propositions.

The validity of such an approach depends on the logic of its conceptual relations and on its basis in an articulated theoretical framework. As Mitchell (1983) has argued, the inferential process involved in extrapolation from individual case studies is one of analysis rather than enumerative induction. (Nevertheless, as he points out, much confusion has arisen because of the misconception that extrapolation from statistical samples can dispense with such logical inference.)

The adoption of a case-study approach here has allowed for an examination in depth and for the cross-referencing of statements. It has been possible not only to compare the views of interviewees in relation to the general issues of this study, but also, more concretely, their views of each other, thus providing an important multi-perspective dimension. Further, it has not been necessary to accept or dismiss the statements of interviewees as either, respectively, universal 'truths' or mere idiosyncrasies. Rather, they have been regarded as opportunities for the critical analysis of the social, political, and economic context which makes such statements both possible and ineluctable. Researchers

do not regard the remarks they collect and typify as constituting some essential truth: they are rather impelling rhetorical statements which, when collectively evaluated, can be seen to derive their persuasive potency – that is, their situational truth – from their context, from the often complex, overlapping, ironic relationships which they bear to other culturally 'true' vocabularies of motive.

(Taylor 1979: 153)

Chapter Two

RULES AND AUTHORITY

> The law in recognizing knowledges beyond itself ...abandons its
> own claim to be the exclusive form of penal discourse.
>
> (Garland 1985: 28)

Magistrates, solicitors, psychiatrists, and probation officers know
about female offenders.[1] They often say they don't, but they act as
though they do. They have to – it is their job. They are authorized
by law to judge, defend, assess, treat, and punish such women and
their occupational·ideologies require that they do so from a base
of privileged understanding. That is not to say that individuals
may not privately or even publicly on occasions deny that
understanding. But such modesty is no more than an apparent
paradox, which requires reconstruction as coherence and
demands action as though understanding existed.

The origin of authority in court is not monolithic. Both
legislatively and conventionally, the roles of the various actors in
the drama have developed in a piecemeal, and at times
conflictual, fashion. Spheres of influence have broadened and
narrowed periodically and inconsistencies both within and
between roles have affected the relationships of power. Legal
parameters at times conflict with notions of professional
judgement and changes in economic or social policy threaten to
turn legal issues into moral and political ones. In the face of this
fragmented and ever-changing reality, how is the legitimacy of
official accounts maintained and protected against the subversion
of the unofficial account – the Other which presages social
disorder and ultimate chaos?

LEGAL RULES

The rights of judicial, medical, and welfare personnel to administer 'criminal justice' are frequently represented as being inherent in the notion of 'natural justice'. There is an assumption that there exists an entity called 'the community' which, although it consists of widely differing interests, can ultimately accommodate those differences in a natural sovereign consensus, which is reflected in the administration of justice rather than being constructed by it. But the rights of these agencies to intervene are neither self-evident nor natural. They do not inhere in any notion of 'citizenship' or 'community'. They are themselves defined and regulated by law. Specialists and experts (which, it will be argued, include 'lay' magistrates) do not possess any natural right to control, supervise, or judge the actions of others, nor do they have unlimited or unfettered competence (or capacity) to do so. 'Law defines the status of the specialist practices and sets limits to the powers of the agents and institutions involved' (Hirst 1980: 92).

But the administration of criminal justice, although defined and regulated by law, must be seen to be to some extent independent of the law, for, in a democratic state, there must be checks and balances to counter the absolutist tendencies of the law-makers. For justice to be seen to be done the law must be seen to be administered by agents who draw their authority from discourses which are 'outside' and therefore beyond the control of the law. Thus they are able to challenge the otherwise unyielding rigidity of the law. For example, doctors are seen to be able to challenge the law's basic premise that all subjects are equally responsible for their actions or equally fit to receive its punishment; social workers are seen to be able to remind the law of its responsibility towards the welfare and rehabilitation of the subject, as well as her punishment; solicitors are seen to be able to preserve the rights of the subject in the face of the seemingly overwhelming assertion of the rights of the state; and, finally, lay magistrates and jurors are seen to be able to safeguard (through 'common sense') the interests of the whole community against the abuse of power by any of the other agents of decision.

Agents are ascribed certain statuses within the court-room, the concept of 'status' consisting of both rights and capacities. The problematic nature of status in magistrates' courts lies in the extent to which experts derive their status from outside the court-room and how that status is structured or restructured within the court-room. What strands of 'knowledge' are sanctioned and what bits are excluded as inappropriate? For example, while a female magistrate may be officially recruited to ensure a balance of the sexes, she may feel herself prohibited from expressing her 'femaleness' in her practice on the Bench (see Chapter 4). Similarly, while a solicitor may recognize the material causes of much crime, the expression of such 'knowledge' is deemed inappropriate to her or his status as a speaker of strictly legal discourse (see Chapter 5). The probation officer, on the other hand, who is allowed to talk of material deprivation, is deemed not to understand the complexities of legal discourse. Thus it is possible, by fragmenting the ascribed rights and capacities of the experts, to ensure the perpetual reproduction of difference and contradiction in a way which renders the challenge to dominant notions of community and consensus ineffective.

GENDER-NEUTRAL JUSTICE?

Carlen (1976) has argued that legal rules are portrayed as being homogeneous, unproblematic, external, inevitable, essential, and eternal. In other words, they are portrayed as 'holding good', over time, across localities, and, more significantly, across the social divisions of class, gender, and race. Legal rules are, therefore, assumed to be gender-neutral and the processing of female law-breakers – with very few exceptions – theoretically unproblematic. Courts do not, therefore, consciously take systematic account of differential circumstances and experiences arising from the social construction of masculinity or femininity. In practice, however, they constantly struggle to reconcile notions of formal gender-neutrality with evidence of substantive gender-inequality in the lives of the women who appear before them. An analysis of the strategies whereby different personnel sustain an appearance of gender-neutrality requires the dismantling of a number of myths which permeate the various occupational ideologies. Those myths and their origins are identified here; their deconstruction comprises the central project of the remainder of this book.

Amateur justice and common sense

I like to think we use our common sense.

(Magistrate 1 – female)

Although the roots of amateur justice go back to the thirteenth-century 'keepers of the peace', the judicial aspect of justices' work did not assume the form that we know today until the nineteenth century, with the passing of the Summary Jurisdiction Act 1848 (Burney 1979). While the purpose of this Act was to formalize and regulate the power of magistrates (for example, by establishing rights of public access and the right of the accused to be represented by a lawyer), the experience of summary justice has come to be characterized by the sacrifice of many of the attributes of the ideology of law, legality, and a fair trial in the interests of speed and efficiency. This sacrifice is usually justified on the grounds that magistrates deal only with 'trivial' matters, but triviality, like beauty, is in the eye of the beholder and may ultimately derive less from the nature of the offences and the penalties of the magistrates' courts than from the triviality in authoritative eyes of the defendants (McBarnet 1981).

Despite this jaundiced view of magistrates' courts as conveyor belts for the guilty pleas that constitute 95 per cent of their case-load, it must be admitted that the appointment of lay magistrates represents an explicit statement about the need to safeguard the interests of 'the community' against the abuse of the power of the law by 'experts', whether those be legal, medical, or social work experts. Summary justice, it may be argued, is not simply a quicker, cheaper form of justice; it has the potential to be a qualitatively different form of justice, for it is concerned with the fundamental tension in a liberal society between 'legality' and 'community'. On the one hand, legality can be seen as providing a basis for co-operative living (and hence a sense of 'community') in a world where there can be no guarantee of shared values. On the other, the personal qualities of the 'decent, honest citizen ... stability, a balanced mentality and common sense' (Burney 1979: 87) are of themselves no guarantee of 'fair' justice, unless that common sense is informed by some understanding of legal rules (Bankowski *et al.* 1987).

So the idealist argument goes. But an alternative analysis might

17

be that the ideology of amateur justice *requires* the absence of legality and that the 'legally informed' common sense which purports to safeguard against the excesses of the experts is little more than thinly disguised privilege – a form of class expertise.

Magistrates appeal to common sense in order to account for their actions. In so doing they make assumptions about 'what everyone knows' to be self-evidently true (i.e. Carlen 1976). They free themselves from any obligation to justify their actions on any other, more 'professional' grounds. By using the term 'common sense' magistrates make their activities 'visibly rational and reportable for all practical purposes' (Garfinkel 1968). They are, as ethnomethodological studies have demonstrated, employing a procedural device which allows them to make sense of data which have no inherent meaning or coherence. They are establishing rules for handling such material and for minimizing any challenge to their handling of it.

One of the central characteristics of common sense is the assumption of a 'reciprocity of perspectives' (Cicourel 1968). As representatives of the community, magistrates take it for granted that most 'ordinary' people would have a similar experience of the immediate scene in question if they were to change places with them. Consensus about law and order issues is something which is assumed to exist among all decent folk, regardless of their gender, age, class, or political allegiance – regardless, in short, of individual difference. Thus represented, common sense becomes the metaphor for those statements which tend to be excluded by experts and which, when uttered, tend to threaten the authority of experts. It consists of all those crude, unrefined, and challenging statements which are unanswerable within expert discourse like those uttered by the magistrate who told me that she and her colleagues 'take psychiatric reports with a pinch of salt'.

Common sense is an elusive and multi-faceted construct, but its unspoken goal is singular – the reproduction of consensus. *Common* sense is sense which is not only common because it is crude but because it is purported to be held universally to be true and to be universally applicable. It is common *sense* not only because it is the opposite of nonsense or falsehood, but because it is 'sensed'. It is truth which is not accessible to rational thought or argument. On the contrary, it is intuitive, instinctive, and accessible only to the senses. It has to be experienced. But this logically detracts from its universalizability, for my experience is unique, as is yours. Yet, despite this acknowledged difference or paradox, its appeal remains in its claim to be stating that which can be recognized by everyone as describing truthfully their own lived experience and which can always and already be inscribed upon the lived experience of others. 'Common-sense has its own necessity; it exacts its due with the weapon appropriate to it, namely, an appeal to the "self-evident" nature of its claims and considerations' (Heidegger 1949, quoted in Carlen 1976: 26).

Common sense may thus be portrayed comfortingly as the safeguard of the criminal justice system, the champion of freedom, the check on expert power. In a democratic society, if justice is no longer majestirial (Hay 1975), then at least it is not dictatorial. Its administration appears to have become a very practical project, a matter of face-to-face interaction and negotiation. The meaning of justice is reduced to the individual consciousness of thousands of actors who daily play the court-room game. Conversely, the abstract concept of justice is perceived as being no more than the aggregate of these atomistic interactions.

But the administration of justice is not a game (Carlen 1976), and the rules governing it are not freely agreed upon by the participants. Certain personnel are given more authority to define than others and certain accounts more credibility than others. The common sense which magistrates claim to be universally recognizable by all citizens is, rather, a specific discourse sanctioned by law and elevated in practice to the status of 'expertise'. In short, majestirial justice has been replaced by magisterial common sense.

Representation and taking instructions

Legal representation in the magistrates' court is not typically a process of defending accused people against their accusers, since, even with representation, the vast majority of defendants appear to plead guilty (Bottoms and McClean 1976). It is rather a process of defending the court against the unacceptability of the layperson's common sense which, unlike magisterial common sense, is perceived to be 'out of place, out of time, out of mind

19

and out of order' (Carlen 1976: 104) and consequently a dangerous intrusion in the proceedings. Representation is therefore a strategy whereby the non-legitimated account (the Other) of the defendant is confronted, controlled, and rendered 'normal'. The common sense of the defendant's account does not accord with magisterial common sense because the latter has been elevated to the status of expertise, whereas the former remains unrecognizable in the court-room. The use of identical vocabulary masks the significant difference of the 'like-us-yet-not-like-us' paradox that indefatigably confronts the magistracy. The role of the solicitor is to occupy that gap between the defendant's account and the magistrates' recognition of that account. The solicitor's task is to negotiate the precise route whereby that gap is closed. It is a task which requires both skill and authority. Solicitors' discourse claims its authority from the precision of the language of statute but 'the general principles of English law are not to be found in the statute book' (Burton and Carlen 1979: 56). The dominant mode of legal reasoning in English courts is that of a 'common law approach', ostensibly characterized by the rigid principle of *'stare decisis'* – the binding authority of precedent. Nevertheless, the law in practice is paradoxically flexible. If legal reasoning were as rigid as the doctrine of precedent suggests, there would be no need for the eloquence and rhetoric of lawyers, for the facts would speak for themselves. Consistency and continuity would be the overriding principles. In reality, 'it is often difficult to be sure just which features of a case were the decisive ones' (Pitkin 1972, quoted in Burton and Carlen 1979: 56). Legal reasoning more commonly seems to be characterized by inconsistency and discontinuity. Some writers have argued from an interactionist perspective (e.g., Bottoms and McClean 1976) that solicitors have the power either to clarify or to fog the law and thus to contribute to or to prevent the negotiation of an ultimately attainable justice, which accords with a form pre-existing in nature (namely, natural justice). Others (e.g., Carlen 1976; McBarnet 1981) have argued that 'justice' is no more and no less than the name we give to that which is (re)produced by the law, within the institution of the law. The power of the solicitor does not lie in some machiavellian skill to distort the 'truth'. Nor does it lie simply in the symbolic interaction between individual solicitor, individual law-breaker, and individual magistrate. The power of the solicitor is institutionalized in the paradox of the common law approach, for s/he theorizes at the interstices of legal rigidity and judicial flexibility. If judges and magistrates see themselves as 'mediat[ing] justice via a legality of which they are the evolutionary embodiment' (Burton and Carlen 1979: 55), then solicitors see their own articulation of legal reasoning as an essential contribution to that process of evolution.

Solicitors' discourse is a self-conscious, spoken discourse – an oral intervention. Its unspoken goal is the 'normalization' of the defendant through a process which packages and re-presents the defendant as a coherent unity which is recognizable by the magistracy. Normalization is the process whereby an illegal action and the person who commits that action are re-presented as 'typical' (Sudnow 1965). The circumstances surrounding the action, the characteristics and motives of its perpetrator, the consequences for the victim, all have to be located within categories that are already known and recognized. Normalization, then, consists of particular practices of inclusion and exclusion, and the skilled task of the solicitor involves anticipating and controlling the variety of possible consequences of these practices. Tacit rules govern these practices but, while these rules are understood by solicitors and magistrates, they are rarely explained to the defendant. First, the defendant is disqualified as speaker – her/his account is muted. Second, certain topics are prohibited or redefined. More specifically, poverty is a prohibited topic because it is a social rather than a legal category. The law does not recognize wealth or its lack as in itself relevant explanation of crime. Magistrates respond to mitigations of poverty with comments such as 'Nobody is poor nowadays' or, alternatively, 'Many people are poor but they don't all turn to crime'. 'Need' is the permitted redefinition of poverty because it implies both relativity (and is thus open to personal interpretation and judgement) and individual inadequacy ('need' is a subjective experience, whereas 'poverty' implies a measure of objective assessment). However, explanations of 'need' cannot be employed where the effect of such an explanation would be to attribute blame to the magistrates, as representatives of the community, or to imply that the alleviation of that need lies within their (or the community's) power.

Although this process of normalization may be directed primarily towards the protection of the court, it is also perceived as a process which protects defendants from themselves and their own natural inclinations to bargain for their liberty even by admitting guilt. 'Uppermost in the mind of the defendant is the urge to freedom, the desire to extricate himself from this uncomfortable situation' (Heberling 1978: 102). Compelled by this 'instinct', few defendants consider the long-term consequences of admissions of guilt and the role of the solicitor as protector is acknowledged, although the practice of 'plea-bargaining' (that is, informally securing promises of sentencing discounts for defendants who initially want to plead 'not guilty') has raised fundamental questions about the nature and justification for legal representation (Bottoms and McClean 1976; Baldwin and McConville 1977).

Nevertheless, all these practices are justified ultimately on the grounds that defendants have *chosen* to engage the services of a solicitor. Contracts have been entered into freely via the fiction of 'giving instructions' and defendants are presented as remaining the knowing subjects/authors of their own discourses. In reality, they have become the objects of another discourse. They have given permission for their statements to be re-iterated according to the rules of solicitors' discourse. They have lost control of their readings, while retaining a faith in the myth of remaining in control.

Solicitors do not talk about making assessments (as, for example, do social workers, probation officers, and doctors); they talk about 'taking instructions'. The implication is that they, as servants, articulate with confidence and competence in public that which the defendant has said nervously and haltingly in private. But what in fact happens is that a privileged discourse is constructed from the broken utterances of the powerless. Discontinuity is rendered continuous, contradiction rendered coherent, and fragmentation rendered unified. A grid is placed over the circumstances and emotions of the defendant and a recognizable reading obtained. In short, an assessment is made.

Having thus assessed the defendant, the solicitor is then required to assess the magistrates whom s/he is addressing. The tacit injunction which governs solicitors' performance was described to me thus by one solicitor:

You get to know your Bench – you play to the audience.

'Getting to know your Bench' involves speculation about the way in which defendants are perceived by magistrates. It involves taking account of magisterial common sense; it also involves taking account of those factors which magistrates themselves deny to be influencing them, but which solicitors recognize all too well as being influential. Those factors – commonly referred to as 'extra-legal' – include class, race, age, political allegiance – and gender.

Consultancy and treatability

Legislation privileges psychiatric discourse at a number of stages in the judicial process[2] and authorizes it to intervene in decisions about both culpability (how responsible was the defendant for her/his actions?) and management (how should s/he be treated?). None of these provisions, however, is mandatory. Ultimately, psychiatrists are no more than expert advisers to the court, whose influence depends on their ability to establish themselves in court more as 'wise men' (Foucault 1965) who have the power to create order out of disorder than as men of science. Psychiatrists are expected to enter into a helpful collusion with the court, passing moral as well as medical judgements on defendants:

> The courts have known me for a very large number of years and, rightly or wrongly, I have a reputation for knowing what I am doing and if I think a person is a villain and there's nothing wrong with him, I say so quite unequivocally.
>
> (Dr A)

Such moral judgements are possible within psychiatric discourse because a) there is no agreement about the nature of mental illness and b) there is no agreement about the relationship between mental illness and criminal activity. Increasingly, when serious crime is at issue (as, for example, in the case of Peter Sutcliffe, the 'Yorkshire Ripper'), courts appear to reject the assertion that 'mental disorder' negates intent to commit a crime, thus placing a question mark over its effectiveness in reducing culpability. Even if a court does accept that a defendant is, by reason of mental disorder, less culpable than otherwise, this does not logically dictate whether s/he should be treated more leniently (because s/he is deserving of sympathy and in need of protection from the full wrath of the law) or more harshly (because s/he is likely to be less amenable to non-punitive measures, dangerous, and in need of control). Consequently, the allocation of 'mentally abnormal offenders' directly to sites of medical jurisdiction is by no means assured. On the contrary, while psychiatric discourse has inseminated the whole of the judicial and penal process (Carlen 1986), its claim to authority emanates as much from its power to exclude defendants from treatment as from its power to admit them to it.

Attitudes to psychiatric discourse among members of the magistracy and the legal profession are ambivalent. Decisions to privilege psychiatric utterances are made on the basis of non-medical factors such as the severity of the offence, personal knowledge of the psychiatrist, and the extent to which the authority of the utterances can be recognized. Psychiatrists are afforded a privileged status within the criminal justice system but they have no right of access to courts. They may speak only at the request of magistrates, solicitors, and probation officers and what they say has to be expressed in a form which is recognizable within the occupational ideologies of those personnel.

One might be tempted to argue that forensic psychiatrists are themselves muted. But psychiatrists are not dependent for their survival and privilege on their recognition by the courts. Their real power derives from elsewhere – from the ideologies and material conditions of medicine and the health services. If courts have the right to reject psychiatrists' statements, then psychiatrists are under no obligation to recognize 'the putative legal subject – s/he, who having (or not) the capacity to know better, breaks the law' (Carlen 1986: 241). Thus, the subject of forensic psychiatry's inquiry is forever elusive. The conditions under which legal subjects are recognized by psychiatry are governed by the rules of *consultancy* – a strategy which perpetuates the myth of the authority of diagnostic input coupled with an absence of responsibility for the consequent outcome. As Nils Christie has said, 'Recently there has been over-emphasis on using medical personnel for the diagnosis stage. A maximum of energy is used for giving advice to the courts and little is left for treatment' (Wolstenholme and O'Connor 1973, quoted in Carlen 1986: 261).

The Mental Health Act 1983 introduced a formal 'treatability' criterion which requires that, before making hospital orders in respect of an offender suffering from psychopathic disorder or mental impairment, a court must be satisfied that medical treatment is 'likely to alleviate or prevent a deterioration of his condition' (s.3). The expressed purpose of this criterion was to prevent the compulsory incarceration of mentally handicapped and other 'abnormal' people simply on the grounds that they were 'abnormal' if they were neither dangerous nor being actively medically treated. It has also been argued that it is wrong to make an offender who is considered untreatable subject to a hospital order, release from which depends on response to treatment (Ashworth and Gostin 1984). The effects of the criterion, however, have been contradictory. The terms 'psychopathic disorder' or 'personality disorder' (the latter normally being seen as a milder version of the former) are supreme examples of this. Since the 'conditions' are considered to be virtually untreatable, the labels are used 'not as a legitimation for intervention but as a ground for declining to intervene' (Allen 1986: 98). They enable psychiatrists to assess and judge, without obliging them to treat. Instead, they are permitted to elevate personal preferences to the status of scientific utterances:

Well some of them are not treatable. You have to decide in terms of age and behaviour and other factors whether there are symptoms that you can modify. With some people who have long-standing personality disorders that have become entrenched and intractable you have to face the fact that there is nothing you can do. This is the general approach to everyone – men and women – you have to be very selective. That's the approach of the new [sic] Mental Health legislation – that they've got to be treatable.

(Dr B)

The formal 'treatability' test applies only to defendants diagnosed as suffering from psychopathic disorder or mental impairment and not to those diagnosed as suffering from other forms of mental illness. However, orders made on the latter are subject to review after six months and only renewed if the defendant's condition is 'treatable'. This has resulted in an informal 'viability' criterion (Ashworth and Gostin 1984), the ideology of which has permeated the diagnosis of all defendants who are referred for psychiatric assessment.

Alternatives to custody and tactical trading

A court may make a probation order for between six months and three years on any adult defendant if it considers that it is 'expedient to do so' and with the defendant's consent. Consent implies a willingness to 'co-operate with his [sic] supervising probation officer as regards reporting, receiving visits and heeding the advice given to him' (Home Office 1986a: 31). Legally, the probation order retains its status as a measure to be used at the court's discretion 'instead of sentencing', although it has been possible, since the 1982 Criminal Justice Act, to appeal against the making of an order. Officially, however, the probation order 'stands outside the normal tariff' (Home Office 1986a: 32). According to Millard (1982), the probation order is (and should continue to be) the mechanism whereby courts can institutionalize their ambivalence (and, by implication, the ambivalence of the community) towards certain offenders. It allows a court to say to a defendant: 'We are uncertain about what you deserve and what you need. Although we cannot be completely merciful with you, we do think you need some kind of help' (Millard 1982: 291). In a 'morally pluralistic' society, Millard argues, where 'no-one is sure any more who ought to be punished and who ought to be helped', the probation order represents an attempt to manage 'the built-in unresolvable tension between the need for repression on the one hand and a commitment to mercy on the other' (1982: 291).

Additionally to the basic condition of a probation order, courts have the power to include requirements of medical treatment, residence (normally at an approved probation hostel), or attendance at a day centre, the purpose of the latter being 'to divert people on probation from a pattern of re-offending by involvement in practical and positive tasks under the supervision of probation staff' (Home Office 1986a: 35).

Courts may also impose a Community Service order of between forty and 240 hours, to be completed within twelve months, on any consenting offender over the age of 16 years, for whom suitable work is available. By requiring the offender to 'perform unpaid work on behalf of the community' (Home Office 1986a: 41), such orders are seen primarily as a means of a) depriving an offender of some liberty in the form of his/her time, and b) exacting some reparation (albeit indirectly) for the harm presumed to have been done to the community by the offender. The measure was initially intended to be a direct 'alternative to custody' (that is, based on the assumption that it is possible to assess by some objective criteria that some offenders, if undiverted, will go to prison).

The involvement of the Probation Service in such orders, however, made it inevitable that 'through subsequent custom and practice, the order has come to be regarded as a sentence in its own right' (Home Office 1986a: 41). The inevitability of this process was due to the ineluctable commitment of traditional probation discourse to the rehabilitation of the offender through the personal influence of the probation officer, which made it difficult for officers to adapt to a role which might be concerned exclusively with the provision and supervision of work. If, as Millard (1982) suggests, this commitment is reinforced by the courts' views of probation officers as people who permit them to be uncertain, it is perhaps not surprising that the Community Service order has become almost as versatile a sentencing option as the probation order.

But probation officers are not merely the passive recipients and administrators of court orders. The history of the Probation Service has been one of increasing influence as sentencing advisers, through the preparation of social inquiry reports.[3] Probation officers prepare such reports after a finding of guilt at the request of the court, though it has always been acceptable for officers to take the initiative in preparing reports if they feel this will be helpful and avoid time-consuming remands, especially if the offender is already known to the Probation Service. In making sentencing recommendations, probation officers are faced with the dual dilemma of defining the appropriate 'moment of intervention' and defining the appropriate 'nature of intervention' in relation to any given potential client. That decision is made as the result of a professional assessment of the relationship between client need, agency resources, and client motivation (that is, the extent to which the client's expressed desire to change is judged by the probation officer to be 'genuine' and the extent to which s/he is judged to have the capacity to benefit from the help available). That assessment must then be translated into

27

language which is 'acceptable' to the court. The defendant must be represented in a form which is recognizable by solicitors, psychiatrists, and, above all, magistrates.

Traditionally, probation officers have claimed authority for such reports on the grounds that they contain recommendations of 'expertly selected treatment based on scientific diagnosis' (Raynor 1985: 153). Nowadays, however, probation officers are more modest in their claims:

> Any opinion expressed in the report about the appropriateness of some form of contractual sentencing ... should be offered to the court as a plausible alternative to the retributive tariff sentence ...The important issues are what the offender is prepared to do, whether and how far the social work agency is able to help him do it, and what assurances the court will require from both parties.
>
> (Raynor 1985: 153)

This dramatic restructuring of the professional ideology of the Probation Service is the result of its emergence in the 1980s from what has been described as its 'loss of direction' in the 1970s (Raynor 1985). Traditional probation work has been forced to accommodate attacks on the 'rehabilitative ideal' from critics of both the political right and left. On the one hand, 'treatment' has been dismissed as little more than 'compulsory persuasion' (Raynor 1978), amplifying rather than reducing deviance. On the other, the apparent desire of 'common sense', hailed by the 'new right', has required that offenders are more strictly supervised and called to account. Such attacks have created tensions for probation officers, from which a sense of 'dissonance' has resulted (Harris 1980).

The banner under which the Probation Service has re-created its identity and restored its self-confidence has been that of 'Alternatives to Custody'. The emphasis in work with offenders has been laid increasingly on negotiation, responsibility, and informed choice (Raynor 1985). Faith is placed in the compelling logic of rational argument to influence both court and client. Clearly, since offenders are held responsible for their actions, they may have to face the fact that their choices are limited and that the nature of their freedom may have to be negotiated with the court. But within this model, such limitations are compatible with the offer of realistic help rather than so-called treatment by experts (Bottoms and McWilliams 1979).

In practice, however, this often means that probation officers are forced to work tactically. In order to get the 'best deal' for their clients in an imperfect judicial world, probation officers may have to compromise their principles of justice and equality, accepting severity in some aspects of sentencing in order to secure leniency in others. Such a process might be described as achieving a 'tactical trade-off' (Garland, 1985: 193). The rules governing tactical trading are paradoxical, for they require the probation officer simultaneously:

a) to recognize (in order to claim authoritative understanding of the offender) and deny (in order to make 'realistic' recommendations to the court) the conditions of social and economic disadvantage in which many offenders exist;

b) to intervene (in order to prevent recidivism) and not to intervene (in order to prevent the amplification of deviance) in the lives of offenders; and

c) to care for the offender (implying an attempt to increase his/her choices in the interest of personal growth) and to control the offender (implying the restriction of choice for the protection of society).

CONCLUSION

Magistrates, solicitors, psychiatrists, and probation officers together constitute a 'chain of signification' in the court-room, authorized to define and give unified meaning to the fragmented and contradictory reality which brings defendants into their purview. They derive that authority from two often conflicting sources:

a) from the law itself, which defines and regulates the rights and capacities of agents to intervene in (and construct) the field of social relations in which subjects move; and

b) from claims to 'expertise' which purport to be independent of the law.

As Garland argues:

Once ...the absolute tenets of the law are opened up to qualifications, the way is open for a continuing struggle between the law and the various human sciences that claim the right to speak on issues of personal character and conduct.

(Garland 1985: 29)

One of the rules governing this struggle is that the exercise of authority should be seen to be *gender-neutral*. The myth of gender-neutrality is sustained and routinely reproduced through adherence to beliefs that magistrates dispense *amateur justice* governed by *common sense*; that solicitors represent clients on the basis of *instructions* received; that psychiatrists offer *consultancy* in relation to the *treatable* and that probation officers *trade tactically* to secure *alternatives to custody*. Within such ideologies, gender (and, indeed, race and class) can be seen to be irrelevant. Yet the routine production of criminal justice is experienced somewhat differently by a significant minority of female law-breakers and by those charged with their care and control.

Chapter Three

NOT MAD ENOUGH, NOT BAD ENOUGH: FIFTEEN FEMALE LAW-BREAKERS

Crime and law enforcement are presently male-dominated worlds and women who enter them threaten the maintenance of the power relationship between men and women (Adler 1987; Edwards 1984; Heidensohn 1985; Smart 1976). Criminality is still assumed to be a masculine attribute and women criminals are therefore perceived to be either 'not women' or 'not criminals'. Many women who break the law also have the attributions of normality which provoke the latter description and thus tacitly collude with attempts to minimize the consequences of their criminality by rehabilitating them within the dominant discourses of femininity.

The female law-breaker is routinely offered the opportunity to neutralize the effects of her law-breaking activity by implicitly entering into a contract whereby she permits her life to be represented primarily in terms of its domestic, sexual, and pathological dimensions (Carlen and Worrall 1987). The effect of this 'gender contract' is to strip her law-breaking of its social, economic, and ideological dimensions in order to minimize its punitive consequences. Many female law-breakers accept this deal; some reject it outright (Carlen *et al.* 1985).

There exists, however, a group of female law-breakers who create particular problems for the criminal justice system because they neither accept nor reject the 'gender contract'. They are the women who are constantly on the margins of categories – never sufficiently this or that – and seeming to defy description. They never seem to be 'dealt with' to the system's satisfaction. Despite (or because of) everyone's best endeavours, they remain 'nondescript' – out of reach and untouchable. The ground on which their relationships are built appears to be shifted constantly within the contradictory discourses

31

of the definers and they seem to frustrate all offers of help and structure. They are women who tend not to assert themselves or to challenge openly, but who use a variety of subterfuges to sabotage attempts to observe, assess, classify, and change them.

It may be argued by some that there exists a similar group of male law-breakers who are persistently resistant to influence. They do not, however, defy description in the same way. On the contrary, the mushrooming provision within the criminal justice system (since the introduction of Community Service in 1972) of 'Alternatives to Custody' has been based on an acknowledgement of the challenge presented by 'persistent petty' male law-breakers. Similarly, current models of juvenile justice (Rutherford 1986) emphasize the normality of adolescent male delinquency and the legitimation of minimal intervention by potentially stigmatizing 'helping' agencies. And, if all else fails, our soaring prison population testifies to the acceptability of dismissing persistent male law-breakers as unmotivated, incorrigible rogues. The nondescript female law-breaker presents a greater moral dilemma, since her ideological (if not her material) positioning at the centre of the family requires that greater efforts be made to rehabilitate her within the discourses of femininity.

There are several reasons why the women on whom this study is based are not, and cannot be presented here as, 'typical' criminal women. First, since they are unclassifiable, they are, by definition, 'untypical' and, second, as Carlen (1985:10) argues, 'there can be no such thing as the "typical" criminal woman'. Third, they may not, in practice, represent the majority of women who commit offences. None the less, the search for 'nondescriptiveness, – the desire to evade the consequences of being seen as a stereotypical woman – is a crucial (and hitherto neglected) element in the activity and behaviour of many female law-breakers. Exploiting the material and ideological conditions that underlie nondescriptiveness is one of the ways in which female law-breakers – and indeed all women – say 'no' to the oppressive nature of stereotypical descriptions and prescriptions. By exploring those conditions which determine both prescriptive descriptions and the restricted range of responses available to women a fuller understanding of women's law-breaking and its relationship to class, race, and gender discrimination will be achieved.

THE GENDER CONTRACT[1]

Women's experiences of 'being female' are mediated by their bodies, their minds, and their social interaction. The discourses within which these experiences are structured are constituted by sets of relationships which cluster around the socially ambiguous status of dependence (Eichenbaum and Orbach 1982). On the one hand, femininity is characterized by self-control and independence. Being a normal woman means coping, caring, nurturing, and sacrificing self-interest to the needs of others. On the other hand, it is characterized by lack of control and dependence. Being a normal woman means needing protection (Hutter and Williams 1981). It means being childlike, incapable, fragile, and capricious.

Approbated motherhood in our society is dependent motherhood within the structure of the nuclear family and responsible, co-operative motherhood within the structure of the welfare state. The normal mother is both economically and emotionally dependent on the father of her child, and it is considered essential to that child's welfare to have two parents *in situ* in the family home (Barrett and McIntosh 1982). 'A mother without a male for support is seen as a social problem' (Calvert 1985).

But the buttressing of the nuclear family does not render it autonomous or impervious to the influence of the state. Rather, the family is seen as an agency of 'supervised reproduction', supported by means of 'contract and tutelage' (Donzelot 1979). The means of obtaining this objective vary with the class of family, but the key site of intervention is always the woman as mother. The offer to the middle-class family is that of a contract, an alliance between the family welfare professionals or 'psy' agents (doctors, psychologists, psychiatrists, and social workers) and the mother. By promoting the mother as educator and medical auxiliary, the state secures its influence over the family, and the mother increases her power within the domestic sphere. But for 'unstructured', 'rejecting', or 'deficient' families the objective must be achieved by different means. It is then the mother herself who requires education and supervision through the medium of social work and psychiatry.

The discourse of domesticity is legitimized by privileged (predominantly male) professionals who are empowered to circumscribe the behaviour of women through alliance or tutelage. Their power is frequently delegated to (predominantly female) semi-professionals (e.g., nurses and social workers), who mediate between them and the women who enter the roles of patient or client. These are the 'wise women' (Heidensohn 1985) who, in addition to translating expert knowledge into common sense for the consumption of the always and already failing woman, also purvey an authoritative role model of normal womanhood (Hutter and Williams 1981).

In addition to the requirement of domestic competence, women's behaviour is further circumscribed by the ideology of female biology as disease, which, like the ideology of the family, has its roots in the Victorian era. Its parameters were defined by the male-dominated medical profession that, in collusion with wealthy, white, middle-class husbands, was vigilant to distinguish the 'silly, self-indulgent, and superstitious' malingerer from the genuinely weak and sickly woman, who needed constant rest and (expensive) medical care (Ehrenreich and English 1973). Interestingly, such distinctions were always less relevant for poor and working-class women, who were conveniently deemed inherently stronger and less in need of lengthy medical treatment anyway. Yet the legacy of such distinctions remains, and the assessment of women's eligibility for medical help constitutes a 'practice of exclusion' both from 'normal' femininity and from 'normal' medicine. Allen (1986) has observed that disturbances arising from women's reproductive cycle – along with those deviations of gender role that have come to be defined as 'personality disorders' (sexual deviance, violence, rejection of family relationships) – have been increasingly marginalized by the medical profession. Since they do not display a 'proper' psychiatric symptomatology, women so categorized are excluded from 'proper' psychiatric treatment and are increasingly defined as requiring social work intervention. Thus, certain women are doubly restricted by being constructed within a discourse of sickness which nevertheless denies them access to the means of health.

The ideology of normal womanhood is mediated to women not only by powerful agents of signification, who claim to have authoritative knowledge about appropriate feminine behaviour, but also through women's own material conditions of existence. The essentially normal woman may not exist, but neither does the universally oppressed woman. Class, race, and age all affect the extent to which women can resist the ideological discourses of femininity and the relative significance of these variables is a question of historical, social, and economic specificity, rather than theoretical debate. It has been argued, for example, that teenage girls find it particularly difficult to fulfil role expectations because adolescent femininity is constructed within two conflicting discourses – adolescence, with its emphasis on change, rebellion, and increasing independence, and femininity, which emphasizes passivity, dependency, and the permanence of relationships (Hudson 1984). The experiences of elderly women who face the major agony of seeing a life long partner sicken and eventually die are at least in part dictated by class differences in sickness and mortality among men (Phillipson 1981) and in financial ability to employ nursing assistance. Similarly, it is theoretically an unresolvable debate whether black women are oppressed more by racism, class, or gender. Lees observes that

> Oppressions based on class, race, religion or region have in common their ability to rely upon and indeed a tendency to strengthen, family and community as forms of solidarity and resistance on the part of the oppressed. Sexual oppression, however, is located within these very institutions. (1986: 95)

The fifteen women in this study were predominantly working-class, poorly educated, and living in conditions of poverty. Most had no income other than Social Security Supplementary Benefit and most, for various reasons, were bringing up children on their own. As women on welfare, they were fairly typical of the 10.7 per cent of families identified by the 1981 General Household Survey as being headed by lone mothers (Family Policy Studies Centre 1984). They were also likely to be 'regarded as deviant (if not criminal) by virtue of their lack of economic and emotional dependence upon a male' (Cook 1987: 28). The material position of such women ensured that they were ill-equipped to resist the ideological pressures of privileged discourse relating to femininity, yet they were, ironically, also uniquely ill-equipped to meet its demands. Consequently, these women found themselves trapped by the moral judgements of professionals, who were also confined by the ideological and material conditions of their jobs. The unspoken 'gender contract' offered to these women, based on assumptions about both willingness and capacity to fulfil mutually agreed obligations, was therefore simultaneously binding yet unfulfillable.

FIFTEEN WOMEN – THE OFFICIAL ACCOUNTS

In the course of interviewing probation officers, thirteen women were identified to me as 'troublesome' women, who might nevertheless be prepared to discuss their experiences of the criminal justice system. Of these thirteen, nine eventually agreed to be interviewed, two refused and two agreed, but failed to keep two pre-arranged appointments. Of the remaining two women, one responded to my letter in a local newspaper and one was interviewed during my visit to a Special Treatment Unit. (Her probation officer was contacted subsequently and interviewed.)

With the exception of Fiona, all the women in this sample were the subjects of Probation Service files. Their biographies had been officially written; they had been assessed and classified, not simply in terms of their law-breaking activity (see Table 3.1) but in an endeavour to 'make sense' of the multitude of 'facts' which constituted their official lives (see Table 3.2). Certain dimensions featured strongly in these official accounts, others were notably absent. Domesticity, sexuality, and pathology were prominent; class and race barely, if at all, mentioned. Again with the exception of Fiona, all the women could be described as 'working-class' and all lived in council-owned accommodation. Only Fiona and Kathy worked full-time. Pauline and Janet had part-time jobs but the rest were unemployed. Yet unemployment and poverty were not features of their official biographies. Racism was totally absent as an issue. Only one woman (Carol) was black and neither she nor her probation officer identified racism as contributing to her situation.[2]

Law-breaking/Deviance

Of the fifteen women, thirteen had at least one previous conviction and eight had several. Such statistics immediately rendered these women difficult to classify, since the 'typical' female law-breaker is a first offender. In 1984, for example, 33 per cent of the 15,000 women on probation on 31 December had no previous convictions, compared with 15 per cent of the 38,000 men on probation (Home Office 1986b). Recidivism is thus regarded as a typically masculine quality and one which raises questions about the 'femininity' of the female law-breaker in the minds of those who deal with her.

Table 3.1 Fifteen women: offences and previous convictions

Name & age	Offence	Sentence	No of pre-cons	Nature of pre-cons
Fiona (21)	Conspiracy to cause GBH	Fine	None	–
Jackie (21)	Motoring & drink-related	Probation s.3	Numerous	Theft Drink-related Prostitution
Eileen (29)	DHSS fraud	Probation	One	Theft
Pauline (30)	Shoplifting	Probation	Several	Shoplifting DHSS fraud
Janet (36)	Deception & Shoplifting	Probation	Several	Shoplifting
Ann (36)	Deception, DHSS fraud & theft of electricity	Prison – voluntary after-care	Several	Burglary Damage
Carol (37)	Shoplifting	Community service	Numerous	Shoplifting
Gwen (38)	Damage	Probation s.3	None	–
Veronica (40)	Shoplifting	Suspended sentence Supervision	Several	Shoplifting Drink-related Assault
Maureen (46)	Theft	Probation	Numerous	Theft
Ivy (58)	Shoplifting	Probation s.3	One	Theft
Kathy (20)	Manslaughter	Probation s.3	One	Deception
Linda (24)	Failed to send child to school	Probation	Several	Theft Burglary Assault
Susan (30)	Shoplifting	Probation s.3	One	Shoplifting
Jean (36)	Child abduction	Prison – voluntary after-care	Numerous	Damage Assault Prostitution

Similarly, although the majority of the offences committed by these women were 'typical' offences of theft (mainly shoplifting) and fraud or deception, a number were not. Maureen's offences were seen as typically feminine:

> Always with Maureen, it's been a case of deception – fiddling DHSS or shoplifting or something like this – and usually the

offences are triggered off by family pressures at home. They get in a mess with their money and budgeting and housekeeping.

(Probation Officer 1 on Maureen)

Linda's offence of failing to send her child to school could be regarded as role-inappropriate (the equivalent, perhaps, of status offences among adolescent girls). Jean's offence of baby-snatching, on the other hand, was regarded as highly 'gender-inappropriate', since 'real' women would never do such an aggressive and uncaring thing. Gwen, Jackie, Fiona, and Kathy had also committed 'unfeminine' offences, since they involved aggressive behaviour which was considered unacceptable in women. For example,

It appeared that she upsets the neighbours and she rants on a bit and she was pretty paranoid and she'd finished up throwing a couple of bricks through her own council house windows. But evidently, it had been a series of problems with the police and they had been almost forced to bring her in.

(Probation Officer 2 on Gwen)

None of the women had received their current sentence for offences related to prostitution, but two had previous convictions for such offences. Four women had previous convictions for burglary, damage, or assault.

The majority (ten) of the women were on probation. Five of that group had conditions attached to their probation orders that they should receive medical treatment although, as will be seen later, the inclusion of such conditions appears to bear little relation to the extent of 'illness' diagnosed. Of the remaining five women, one had had no involvement with the Probation Service beyond the preparation of a report for court (Fiona). Three had been on probation in the past but were currently experiencing different forms of contact with their probation officers (Ann, Veronica, and Jean). One (Janet) was serving both probation and a Community Service Order (imposed at two separate but chronologically close court appearances). Carol had a history of contact with the Probation Service but had not actually been on probation in the preceding ten years. She was currently serving a Community Service Order.

Table 3.2 Fifteen women: dimensions of law-breaking

Name & age	Law-breaking/deviance	Domesticity	Sexuality	Pathology	Consequences
Responders					
Fiona (21)	Conspiracy to cause GBH. No previous convictions.	Single, living at home, father dies. 'Good daughter.'	Offence committed in a group with men – under their influence?	'Depression'/fear of discovery by parents /guilt re father's death/remorse.	Crown Court trial; 'lenient' sentence of £100 fine.
Jackie (21)	Numerous motoring and drink-related offences. Long record. In care 12–16 for truancy and theft.	Married with one child. Husband in prison for assaulting her.	Admitted prostitute. 'Promiscuous.'	Assessed as 'personality disorder'.	Placed on probation with condition of in-patient treatment at Special Treatment Unit.
Eileen (29)	DHSS fraud. 1 previous conviction but known to probation and social services since 14 when parents divorced.	Married 3 times 4 children subject to matrimonial supervision – 1 with grandmother, 3 on 'At Risk' register. 'Suspect mother.' Husband in prison.	Unwise choice of partners. Beaten by husband. 'Promiscuous?'	History of 'attention-seeking' overdosing, treatment for 'personality disorder'	Placed on probation for 2 years.
Pauline (30)	Theft (shoplifting). Several previous convictions for shoplifting and DHSS fraud. 2 previous probation orders.	Divorced ('innocent victim'). Two children. 'Good mother.' Lonely, isolated.	'Intelligent lady.' Inadequate husband. Offences seen as expression of sexuality.	Assessed as needing group psychotherapy for 'guilt complex'.	Placed on probation. Attends and enjoys.

Table 3.2 cont.

Name & age	Law-breaking/deviance	Domesticity	Sexuality	Pathology	Consequences
Janet (36)	Deception & theft. Several previous convictions.	Married with 3 children. 'Respectable' but with possible marital problems.	Offences committed in context of 'normal' feminine conduct – i.e., selling hampers, shopping. But 2nd offence seen as 'defiance' (i.e., not feminine).	Referred by PO for psychiatric treatment	Probation for deception but Community Service as 'alternative' to custody' for theft.
Ann (36)	Forged prescription, broke into meter, DHSS fraud. Previous convictions include burglary, damage.	Married with one child (not husband's) in Care. Husband has record. 'Inadequate mother.' Massive debts – won't accept help.	Both she and husband aggressive when drunk. Prostitutes. 'Hasn't reached rock bottom yet.'	Drug and alcohol problem. Won't accept treatment.	Initially placed on probation but breached conditions. Suspended sentence, then prison – prefers prison to hospital.
Carol (37)	Theft. Long record including prison.	Separated. Four children who go into Care when Carol is in prison.	Unwise choices of partner. Cohabits with violent men.	No psychiatric referral. Sees self as stealing by compulsion.	Perceived as professional'. Given Community Service.
Gwen (38)	Damage to own (council) property. No previous convictions.	Single. One child in Care.	Unmarried, without support/control of man.	History of psychiatric treatment.	Narrowly avoided remand in custody. Remanded to hospital. Probation with condition of in-patient treatment.
Veronica (40)	Theft. Previous breach of probation. Several previous convictions, including assault on husband.	Divorced with two children. 'Suspect mother.'	Alcohol problems. Lacking male support.	'Psychopathic personality disorder with excessive drinking habits.'	Crown Court; Suspended Sentence Supervision Order.

Table 3.2 cont.

Name & age	Law-breaking/ deviance	Domesticity	Sexuality	Pathology	Consequences
Maureen (46)	Theft. Long record including prison.	Married but frequently separated. Family now grown up but in Care in the past. '4 very disturbed children.' 'Inadequate mother'	Aggressive & unmanageable but also victim of husband's abuse.	Long history of poor physical and mental health. Multiple diagnoses, including 'personality disorder'.	Probation – no feasible alternative.
Ivy (58)	Theft of jar of coffee. One previous conviction many years earlier.	Divorced, grown-up children all away from home. Lonely, isolated.	Unfaithful to husband. Lacking support/controlling influence of man.	History of psychiatric treatment but 'too lucid' in court	Placed on probation for 3 years with conditions of out-patient treatment.
Non-responders					
Kathy (20)	Killed sister – murder reduced to manslaughter. One previous conviction for minor deception.	Single, lived with family. 'Good daughter.' 'Normal' teenager	Unwise choice of boyfriend. Sister tried to persuade her to give him up – K. stabbed her.	Suspected epilepsy.	Probation with condition of treatment but never seen. 'A tragic case.'
Linda (24)	Failed to send child to school. Previous convictions for burglary, theft, and assault.	Single with 2 children. Recently moved from parents' to own house. Had been 'problem' teenager.	Lacking support/ control of a man.	As a teenager was school phobic, attempted suicide, temper tantrums. In-patient treatment	Probation with 'psy' complex involvement – social services and Education Welfare.
Susan (30)	Shoplifting. One previous conviction.	Divorced and remarried. Child in Care in the past but home now.	Very conscious of weight. 'Attracted' violent, drinking men.	Anorexic? Phobic anxiety, depression, agoraphobia.	Probation with condition of treatment.
Jean (36)	Baby-snatching. Previous convictions for damage, violence, and prostitution. Prison.	Married but separated. 4 children in and out of Care. Has abandoned children on occasions. 'Bad mother.'	Has engaged in prostitution. 'Deprived and undersocialized.' Erratic, violent, etc.	Psychopathic personality disorder, not amenable to treatment, and not mentally ill.	Two-year prison sentence – appeal failed – not granted parole. On voluntary after-care.

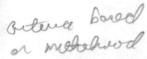

Domesticity

The ages of the women ranged from 20 to 58 years and only the two youngest (Kathy and Fiona) were not mothers. Of the remaining thirteen, only three had failed to attract the tutelary gaze (Donzelot 1979) of the 'psy' agencies in relation to the quality of their mothering. Ivy's children were already grown up and had left home when she committed her offence; Pauline and Janet were considered 'good' mothers. Ten of the mother, however, either had children currently in the care of the local authority (Ann, Gwen, Jean), had had children in Care in the past (Maureen, Carol, Susan) or were under suspicion of being 'bad' mothers (Eileen, Veronica, Jackie, Linda). Jackie and Linda had both been threatened directly with the removal of their children unless they resolved their problems. For Linda,

> the problem does appear to lie with her lack of organization of herself and her family, to make sure that David does attend school on a regular basis.
>
> (Social inquiry report on Linda)

Among other things, she was instructed,

> to seek psychiatric and medical help with her personality disorder in an attempt to organize her own life and thus provide a secure and stable home for her children.
>
> (Case conference notes)

Jackie's problem was excessive drinking and promiscuity. Her psychiatric report contained the following comments:

> Failure to co-operate with our treatment which includes aversion treatment to alcohol followed by regular Antabuse treatment will constitute a breach of the terms of probation....She has been told that unless she does something about the problem, she will jeopardize the chances of keeping custody of her daughter.

Her probation officer (3) informed me:

> That was put in for the sake of the magistrates who were clearly thinking of sending her to prison, and he [the psychiatrist] was very aware of that.

Here, Jackie's status as mother is simultaneously hailed (to compensate for her abnormal sexuality) and denied to enable her to be described within psychiatric discourse as a judicially recognizable subject, in need of both treatment and punishment. Eileen had been under suspicion for a long time:

> We've always had our doubts ...and we had a conference recently ...we were imagining all sorts of things ... we had to look into it. Some of them could probably be substantiated but they're not sufficiently bad to warrant serious action ...I think more than anything those kids will suffer more mentally than physically.
>
> (Probation Officer 4 on Eileen)

The suspect nature of the women's mothering was exacerbated by their suspect 'wifeliness'. Only one woman (Janet) could be considered 'normal' in the sense that she was still living with her first husband, who was the father of her children, and even *her* marriage was seen as possibly contributing to her offences, according to her probation officer:

> One of the things I think we ought to be looking at fairly closely is Mrs T's marriage. Sometimes I tell her off because I don't think we're looking at the questions behind her depression.
>
> (Probation Officer 5 on Janet)

Maureen's marriage, though long-standing, was highly unstable. She had left her husband on numerous occasions. Her psychiatrist was

> more convinced every day that her problem is basically a marital one. I think that, as a psychiatrist, I have very little to offer this lady. Most of her problems are social ones.
>
> (Psychiatrist on Maureen)

Three other women (Jean, Ann, and Jackie) were currently married to their first husbands but all three men also had criminal records. Ann's and Jackie's husbands had been to prison for assaulting them; Jean's husband also abused her when he was drunk. Susan was married for a second time, apparently to a man who was, according to her probation officer, 'much more enlightened'. Her first husband, however,

used to beat her and drink a lot, and made all the decisions
and had quite an old-fashioned view of marriage.

(Probation Officer 6 on Susan)

It had been during this marriage that her child had been taken
into Care. Eileen had been married three times and her present
husband was currently in prison, having been 'shopped' by her. He
had threatened to divorce her and apply for custody of the children
but Eileen was planning for a reconciliation on his release.

Three of the women (Ivy, Veronica, and Pauline) were
divorced. Pauline was viewed by her probation officer as the
innocent victim of an 'inadequate' man who had an affair with
another woman while working away in Scotland.

Then he brought this woman home to meet his wife, and she
was ringing when he came home at weekends – all this sort of
thing she had to cope with. He really did show how inadequate
he was, because he couldn't make the break but he couldn't
decide to stay with his wife.

(Probation Officer 7 on Pauline)

Ivy, on the other hand, received somewhat less sympathy. Her
husband also left her for another *woman*), but her own unfaithfulness
was seen as contributing to the break-up of the marriage. Veronica
was certainly not viewed as an innocent victim, since she had a
history of assaulting her husband when she was drunk.

The remaining three mothers (Carol, Linda, and Gwen) might
well have been defined as bad wives (or even bad women), since
they were not wives but should have been. Carol was separated
and cohabiting with a man who was not the father of all her
children, while Linda and Gwen had never lived with the fathers
of their children.

The two women without children were assessed as daughters.
Fiona and Kathy (despite killing her sister) were both perceived
as 'good, dutiful daughters', living at home and being portrayed
as 'normal' teenagers.

Sexuality

The extent to which these women were deemed to have made
'unwise' choices in relation to men was implicit in discussion of

their domestic situations. It was also, however, an independent theme underlying most of their official biographies. At one extreme, Pauline's plight was described as

> a very sad history of a very inadequate man and a very adequate lady who then decided to become inadequate so that she didn't overshadow her husband.
>
> (Probation Officer 7 on Pauline)

Kathy, too, had been taken advantage of by a feckless man:

> Her feelings for this man were so strong that they blinded her to reality....Everyone could see that this man was simply using her, except Kathy herself.
>
> (Social inquiry report on Kathy)

Carol, Ann, Jackie, and Susan were all seen as 'attracting' men who drank heavily and were violent, the implication being that such men met psycho-sexual needs in them. Jackie's probation officer described her relationship with her husband.

> He'll black both her eyes and walk out. She's very capable of winding him up and he didn't strike me as being a particularly nice character.
>
> (Probation Officer 3 on Jackie)

Three of the women (Eileen, Jean, and Jackie) were described as promiscuous. According to her probation officer, Eileen had a reputation for having numerous boyfriends and this was seen to be antithetical to the welfare of her children:

> She's that sort of girl ...she loves her children, she doesn't want them to go away ...but she's got needs of her own which are far away from the needs of the children really.
>
> (Probation Officer 4 on Eileen)

It was assumed that a woman who attended to her own sexual needs must therefore be either neglectful of the needs of her children or else be placing them in 'moral danger' through her own bad example.

Jackie's probation officer recounts a confrontation between her and her psychiatrist:

By this time she'd been pretty worked up. The doctor told her that she was an easy lay for a drink. I suppose that's fairly accurate, but I suppose she's not used to being talked to like that.

(Probation Officer 3 on Jackie)

One might question the medical status of the psychiatrist's assessment of Jackie but, as will be seen in Chapter 6, 'forensic psychiatry is authoritatively charged with the legal, judicial and *moral* management of law-breakers' (Carlen 1986: 241, emphasis added). Additionally, as white, middle-class professional men, psychiatrists are, within capitalist patriarchal society, ascribed the right to exercise both verbal and physical control over working-class women (cf. Messerschmidt 1987).

Jean's promiscuity dated back to her adolescence, according to her probation records:

Went out every night and became 'lad mad' – says she was described as the 'sex bomb of the estate'... highly promiscuous at the time and this was encouraged by her fellow workers. Confided in older women. The way in which she kept the older women interested was to tell her exploits and this increased her need to engage in such exploits.

(Social history on Jean)

More recently, however, her promiscuity was seen as a form of revenge of her husband:

During her husband's imprisonment, Mrs M prostituted herself and although there was some financial gain, the reason seems to have been anger with her husband, projected on to the men concerned, for whom she had no feelings.

(Social history on Jean)

In committing their offences, whether these women were seen as either too much influenced by men or too little influenced, they were always seen in relation to men. Fiona's offence was committed in a group, most of whom were men. Her lenient sentence may well have reflected a feeling that, as the driver of the 'getaway' car, she had not been directly involved in the assault, but had been under the influence of her male companions. Ann and Maureen were both perceived to be aggressive and unmanageable, but their behaviour was aggravated by the aggression and drinking

46

of their husbands. Gwen, Linda, Veronica, and Ivy, on the other hand, were seen to be in need of supervision because they lacked male support (and, by implication, male control) (see Eaton 1987 on bail decisions relating to women in magistrates' courts).

Pathology

Thirteen of the fifteen women had had some involvement with psychiatrists, although only five had conditions of treatment written into their probation orders. Very little attention was given in the official accounts to the gynaecological dysfunctions referred to earlier in this chapter and such lack of concern appears to reinforce theories that working-class women do not have the same access to the excusing condition of 'inherent fragility' as do their middle-class sisters (cf. Ehrenreich and English 1973; Edwards 1981). Much greater concern was shown about the 'genuineness' of the women's claims to sickness and this concern was buttressed by the elastic nature of the definition of the 'disturbance' invoked (see Chapter 6). As I have argued elsewhere (Worrall 1978), the vaguer that definition, the more likely it is that the 'incongruity' between 'womanhood' and 'criminal-ness' will be maintained. Pauline, for example, was not suffering from any clearly definable mental illness at all, yet, as we shall see, she had greater access to the excusing condition of pathology than any of the women – possibly because she was intelligent, articulate, personable, and potentially middle-class.

One woman who received little sympathy, despite having been hospitalized for anxiety and depression, was Ivy. She pleaded not guilty to stealing a jar of coffee on the grounds that she was confused as a result of recent ECT and drug therapy. Unfortunately, however, she presented herself in court as being extremely clear and lucid, so that she failed to convince the magistrates of her innocence. Ivy's attempt to medicalize her own condition was negated by her failure to present herself as 'muted'. She had been *too* articulate and competent and, ironically, had thus discredited the very defence of her actions she was attempting to make. The trivial nature of her offence also seemed to reinforce rather than reduce her perceived responsibility for her actions. Had she, like Kathy, killed someone, the situation might have been different.

Kathy killed her sister, by stabbing her with a kitchen knife. Yet Kathy, like Ivy, was placed on probation for three years with the condition that she receive psychiatric treatment. Kathy was originally charged with murder but under psychiatric examination it emerged that she may have had a history of epilepsy. It is worth quoting in detail from the report prepared to illustrate the effectiveness of psychiatric discourse in rendering violent women harmless (Allen 1987 a):

> The circumstances of the offence are unusual. K attacked her sister, whom usually she is very fond of. There does not seem to be any obvious motive for the fierceness of the assault. Her behaviour before the act and shortly after it seems to have been relatively unremarkable. K's family describe her as a pleasant young woman and certainly our observations of her while she was here was of a well-behaved, pleasant woman. I understand that, while on bail, she has resumed her job. Her EEG is abnormal. It is indicative of instability rather than frank epilepsy. Instability of an EEG can occur in the absence of epilepsy and can occur in about 50 per cent of normal persons, but unstable records tend to be found in young women of K's temperament and level of immaturity. However, the instability in this case is so marked and is considerably accentuated by the consumption of alcohol. Instability of an EEG often correlates with an aggressive and violent behaviour. On balance, therefore, taking into account K's previous personality, the absence of any comparable assaults, the suddenness and severity of the assault, the lack of any obvious motive, her markedly abnormal EEG, which is accentuated by alcohol, I feel at the material time, she was suffering from such abnormality of mind as would substantially diminish her responsibility for her act and bring her, therefore, within the Section 2 of the Homicide Act 1957.

The charge was reduced to one of manslaughter and, in passing sentence, the judge said to Kathy:

> I'm not going to dwell on the facts. This has been a great burden to you. This is not a case for punishment. Everything possible must be done to help you in the future.

> (Probation file on Kathy)

Following her conviction, Kathy had no contact whatsoever with

Dr A despite his agreement in court to treat her. Two years later, her probation officer (not the original one) wrote:

> K asked me about the question of Dr A and his lack of contact and I suggested that, as there had been no contact with Dr A for so long now, it was pointless to try and resume contact with him. That is, unless K particularly wanted to see him for any reason. Clearly K was not keen to follow anything up in the psychiatric treatment area and I was quite happy to go along with this. I tried to relieve K's anxieties on this question by suggesting that any initiative with regards to treatment would have been made by Dr A in the past and presumably he sees no reason to continue contact with K. K was quite happy with this explanation and feels that she has no need whatsoever to see Dr A at the time.

Psychiatric discourse had, it seems, enabled Kathy to get away with murder, while Ivy continued to receive ECT for stealing a jar of coffee. The reason for this, as Allen also argues (1987a), is that Kathy's crime was so incongruous with her status as a 'very typical teenager' (Social Inquiry Report) that her status as the responsible author of her crime had to be revoked. She had to be presented as not intending and not understanding the consequences of her action. The alternative explanation – namely, that a hard-working, respectable family (according to the SIR) had produced a fratricide – was unthinkable. Yet, in terms of management, Kathy presented the court with few problems, for that same family could be trusted to control and contain her with the minimum of outside intervention. Ivy, on the other hand, was more problematic for, despite the trivial nature of her crime, there was a congruity about her (albeit petty) criminality which indicated the presence of agency (i.e., responsibility). Her social status as a divorcee also suggested an absence of familial control over her behaviour. In her case, therefore, psychiatry was employed not to reduce culpability but to ensure management, suggesting that the criminal justice system is more concerned with the maintenance of social order than with the retributive punishment of crime.

The remaining women exhibited a variety of 'symptoms' which had been broadly classified into two categories, depending on the profession's perception of their 'genuineness'. Pauline, Susan, and

49

Janet were all diagnosed as suffering in some way from anxiety or depression. All three were seen as co-operative and amenable to treatment. Pauline, in particular, was regarded as a 'rewarding' case:

> She's a good person to work with, very intelligent and you can reason things through with her – it's one of those cases where you can put your theory into practice – it's quite good for me.
>
> (Probation Officer 7 on Pauline)

The remaining women were described more negatively as 'attention-seeking', 'manipulative', 'psychopathic', and/or as having 'personality disorders', in some cases exacerbated by 'excessive drinking habits'. Some, like Gwen, Veronica, Eileen, and Maureen, had long histories of psychiatric treatment which was deemed to have 'failed' and they were retrospectively reassessed as 'malingerers'. Others, like Ann, Jean, Linda, and Jackie, were seen as not amenable to conventional treatment, although Jackie was considered suitable for a Special Treatment Unit. According to her probation officer,

> She created and called Dr G this, that and the other and threatened to kill me. And they said 'This girl – she's perfect material for this Unit'!
>
> (Probation Officer 3 on Jackie)

As Dr A remarked, treatment of people with personality disorder 'has to be undertaken by enthusiasts.'

MISCONSTRUCTING THEM AS DOMESTICATED, FEMININE, AND SICK?

It is evident from these official accounts that the routine practice of classifying and describing female law-breakers in particular ways has proved inadequate in relation to the women in this study in providing either explanations of their past law-breaking activity or management of their future behaviour. Far from demonstrating that they are domesticated, feminine, and sick, these women have evaded (often by their sheer passivity) the controlling effects of such categorization. They have presented themselves variously as:

a) suspect or non-mothers and failed wives;

b) sexually indiscriminate and promiscuous women, unsupported and uncontrolled (or uncontrollable?);

c) not mad enough or too mad, alcoholic and malingering.

Yet none of these women would be described as 'villains' (cf. Carlen *et al.* 1985) either. Nor would they be seen as being committed ideologically to protesting against capitalism or patriarchy. They appear to live very mundane lives – some seeing themselves as more 'respectable' than others, some more angry than others, and all of them struggling in relative poverty.

Chapter Four

INVISIBLE WOMEN?

Magisterial common sense is characterized by a denial of expertise coupled with a claim to authority for statements which are assumed to reflect public moral consensus. Despite explicitly disclaiming any legal, medical, or sociological understanding of crime, magistrates implicitly draw selectively from all these and other perspectives in the construction of their own privileged discourse. It is a discourse within which three key myths may be identified as having important consequences for women defendants:

1) Through the process of *self-disqualification* magistrates simultaneously deny and claim authority for what they say; the consequence for women defendants is that they are rendered always and already invisible, inaccessible, and unknowable (yet forever known).

2) Through the invocation of the ostensibly gender-neutral concept of *individual merit* magistrates simultaneously generalize and deny the possibility of generalization; the consequence for women defendants is that they are rendered *intractably heterogeneous*.

3) Through the *privileging of personal life experience* magistrates simultaneously claim and deny similarity with defendants; the consequence for women defendants is that they are rendered *like-yet-not-like women magistrates*.

SELF-DISQUALIFICATION AND THE INVISIBLE WOMAN DEFENDANT

I've dealt with very few women.

(Magistrate 2 – female)

Although women still constitute a small proportion of all defendants appearing in courts, I found only one magistrate who was
aware of any increase in their numbers of recent years. On the
whole, it still seems to be women defendants' scarcity that
characterizes their image in the minds of magistrates – they are
under-represented. It is hard to believe, for example, that the
following statement by a woman magistrate could possibly be
factually accurate:

> I've been a magistrate for ten years and I think I've only had
> three or four women appearing before me.
>
> (Magistrate 3 – female)

Other magistrates were less extreme in their estimates but, as Pat
Carlen (1983) found in Glasgow, most prefaced their remarks
with disclaimers:

> I'm not very helpful on women, I'm afraid.
>
> (Magistrate 4 with 18 years' experience – female)

> For some unknown, unexplained reason, my personal dealings
> with female offenders have been extremely limited.
>
> (Magistrate 5 – male)

Nine out of the twelve magistrates interviewed explicitly
disqualified themselves from being competent to speak about
women defendants. Those with relatively few years' service felt
they lacked experience, while those with longer service implied
that women defendants were too few to justify generalization
anyway. Thus it was made clear that whatever view might
subsequently be expressed by the interviewee, these were based
on no more than anecdotal evidence and were emphatically not
to be taken as authoritative statements.

So the first manifestation of magisterial common sense in
relation to women defendants is an expressed emphasis on self-
disqualification, consequent on perceived lack of experience.
That lack of experience results from limited time in the job ('I've
only been doing this work for five years'), limited access to the
material being studied ('I deal mainly with juveniles and
domestics'), or the elusiveness of such material ('We don't see
many women here'). In other words, women defendants are not

recognized by magistrates because they are invisible. Alternatively, it might be argued that women defendants are invisible to magistrates because they are not recognized as being 'real' criminals. Women are 'out of place' in court (Worrall 1981) and are routinely 'not seen'. Those who do draw attention to themselves as a result of 'unusual' offences, behaviour, or personal circumstances are always and already marked out as 'unfeminine'.

INDIVIDUAL MERIT AND THE INTRACTABLY HETEROGENEOUS WOMAN DEFENDANT

You can't generalize – every case must be treated on its own merit.

(Magistrate 6 – male)

In my opinion, it is important to stress that every case brought before a magistrate is different, due to the circumstances and background of the defendant, whether they are male or female. I believe that my judgement is based much more on the individual rather than their sex.

(Magistrate 7 – female)

Every case is treated on its own merit – it's such an individual thing.

(Magistrate 2 – female)

Every case is treated individually and can never be generalized ....I would again stress that every case must be treated on its own merit.

(Magistrate 8 – female)

Since so few are 'seen' by them, it follows that magistrates claim to be wary of generalizing about women as a category of defendants. A further contribution to this caution is made by the sentencing principle of individualized justice (Edwards 1984; Pearson 1976). The practice of seeking the most suitable sentence for a particular defendant has the effect of depoliticizing the personal circumstances of those appearing in court. This effect becomes exaggerated in relation to women, since, as has been seen in

Chapter 3, femininity is constructed within the private and personal confines of domesticity, sexuality, and pathology. Even when women defendants are 'seen', they are not recognized as sharing, or having in common, any conditions of existence that might explain their law-breaking activity – they are rendered intractably heterogeneous.

The process of individualization is ostensibly gender-neutral but serves, in practice, to reinforce gender distinctions. If each case is treated on its own merits – so the argument goes – it is not possible to generalize on the grounds of age, class, education, or any other socio-economic factor, including gender. Yet this is precisely what magistrates do. Despite their denials, they do demonstrate a sociological understanding of women's position in society and of the stereotypical role expectations of women as wives and mothers. Some magistrates are conscious of the oppressive nature of such role expectations but they are also conscious of the contradictions between this sociological understanding and the formal gender-blindness of the law. The law does not allow for the *social* construction of *legal* subjects. In order to reconcile the contradictions between legal and social construction, the *moral* concept of *merit* is invoked. The appeal to merit is one which is seen to supersede these contradictions, for it is an appeal to the discourse of morality – of right and wrong, good and bad. These are truths which are held to be self-evident. Whether a defendant is a man or a woman, it is assumed that the qualities of goodness and badness, the notions of culpability and mitigation, free-will and determination are also gender-blind. Moral attributes, such as selfishness, callousness, responsibleness, and consideration, are deemed to be universally recognizable and consensually definable. But the concept of 'merit' is itself socially constructed within the ideologies of what constitutes 'meritorious' conduct and these ideologies are themselves gender-related. What is seen to constitute selfish and irresponsible behaviour in a man differs widely from what is seen to constitute such behaviour in a woman. The differential tolerance of drunkenness in men and women is but one example of this (Otto 1981).

Magistrates, in common with the rest of us, are faced with the problem of induction – how and when to move from specific to general statements. The problem is exacerbated, however, because they feel expressly discouraged from using theory to bridge that gap or to redefine the problem as being one of *deduction*. The construct of 'individual merit' allows generalizations to be made at precisely the same time as the possibility of their being made is denied. It provides the means whereby magistrates can reconcile (or close the gap between) the specificity of their own personal experience and the demands of their role. It enables them to act and speak in ways which are just and equitable – that is, generalizable. Thus the individualized, or intractably heterogeneous, woman defendant is a myth, for, despite their denials, magistrates routinely generalize about the women who appear before them.

PRIVILEGING PERSONAL LIFE EXPERIENCE AND THE FEMININE WOMAN DEFENDANT

I feel sad to see a woman in the dock, but I put it out of my mind.

(Magistrate 6 – male)

I do find difficulties in this area. The appearance of a woman in court still upsets me a little....I have to force myself to take an objective view, which I admit would come much more easily when trying a male offender.

(Magistrate 7 – female)

Closely linked to the construct of 'individual merit' – indeed, it may be seen as the opposite side of the same coin – is the mechanism of 'privileging personal life experience'. Magistrates are encouraged to regard their own life experience as 'privileged' in the sense that they are expected to draw on their own experience to inform their judgements. Thus their own personal life experience is ascribed special status within the court-room when the personal life experiences of other personnel are considered irrelevant to the task in hand.

Most magistrates were only too aware of the dilemmas posed by this expectation that they were like-yet-not-like the defendants with whom they dealt and they felt under an obligation to 'make sense' of their practices. Some (both male and female) admitted feeling personally distressed by women defendants but felt obliged to suppress that instinctive response. One magistrate implied that her own personal problems might have resulted in her responding sympathetically to such women but she added, 'I can switch off when I go into court'. The irony of such comments is that, while magistrates are exhorted to use their common sense and trust their intuition (conditioned, as it must be, by their life experience), certain responses, nevertheless, have to be excluded, controlled, or modified in the search for 'objectivity'. Thus 'objectivity', which in most discourses would be taken of necessity to include logical, rational argument and to exclude sensation, is somehow accommodated within magisterial common sense, without posing a threat to it. This is possible because what is being spoken of is not, in fact, objectivity but consensus. What magistrates felt the need to suppress were those responses which they perceived to be unacceptable to their colleagues. They were the responses which might detract from or threaten consensus.

The privileging of personal life experience also allows magistrates legitimately to challenge the assessments of those engaged in professional discourses – to act as the Other intruding into the claims of sovereign knowledge (although, as I have already asserted, this act is a masquerade, for magisterial common sense is itself a discourse). Nevertheless, magistrates are conscious of their power:

> I sit two weeks out of three on Wednesdays – I don't like
> playing God too often.
>
> (Magistrate 1 – female)

She was alone in expressing reservations about this aspect of the role, and another magistrate argued that :

> One is very dependent on the information one is given, or is
> revealed, at the time of trial.
>
> (Magistrate 8 – female)

thus implying a certain powerlessness. Again, magisterial common sense allows for the reconciliation of such a contradiction – the simultaneous exercise of power and its denial. It is not therefore surprising that professional discourse – in particular, psychiatric and social work – met with inconsistent responses. Dependence on reports which buttress common sense discourse was acknowledged:

I do appreciate a good overall report, physical, intellectual, emotional, and social. I have found that well-written, in-depth reports can help tremendously when considering sentence.

(Magistrate 7 – female)

Psychiatric reports which comfortingly reassure magistrates that 'normal' women do not commit crime, and which conveniently reduce criminal activity to female biology are welcomed:

I would expect that *psychiatric reports* would be of great help in sentencing women, due to the points I have mentioned (about strains and tensions of family life). Also, to the health problems which are *particularly relevant to being a female.* In saying this, however, these reports and social inquiry reports are of great value in both men and women.

(Magistrate 3 – female)

But the right to view the quality of that information through the filter of magisterial common sense was considered the magistrates' privilege and reports which challenged such a right were likely to be dismissed. The merits or demerits of such information appeared to be assessed according to a) personal knowledge of the author (cf. Carlen 1976) and b) the extent to which the authority of the utterances could be recognized or, as Edwards puts it, the 'correct anticipation of "observers' rules"' (1984: 145). Thus experts may be ignored if they sound either insufficiently or excessively 'expert':

We take psychiatric reports with a pinch of salt – we have to accept that they are the experts, but some of the things they say are a bit way out – we use our common sense.

(Magistrate 2 – female)

As June Huntington says:

Even when an occupation has a relatively undisputed 'authority to know' its claims may still be weak because the public denies any need for that particular area of knowing. This would appear to be the case with psychiatry.

(1981: 74)

Probation officers may be ignored if they appear too sympathetic towards the defendant and thus fail to meet the requirement for all court-room personnel to appear to be judicious:

> We find that probation officers sometimes bend over backwards towards a defendant – we don't always follow their recommendations.

> (Magistrate 2 – female)

But personal acquaintance is very important.

> Social inquiry reports are excellent from probation officers – and social workers. But social workers don't give verbal evidence well. We get to know probation officers – we need to get to know social workers.
>
> Psychiatrists – I know AA and BB is a close friend, so I trust them. But some from X – well, CC always talked about sex – it was ridiculous. I don't know DD, but she made a bad impression on magistrates early on. She seemed drunk – but she couldn't have been, in her position.

> (Magistrate 4 – female)

It is essential that both reports and their authors are, therefore, (re)presented in a recognizable way:

> Some magistrates don't like being told what to do in reports – there are ways of putting things.

> (Magistrate 4)

Telling a magistrate what to do has the appearance of detracting from the dignity or 'majesty' of the law and reducing the process to one of personal conflict. But discovering the rules which will guarantee the authority of the object of professional discourse to this particular readership is a formidable task, for the very ground on which such rules should be based is constantly shifting. To 'each case on its own merit' might well be added, 'each report received according to taste'. But is the process quite so unpredictable and arbitrary?

The strategy employed by magistrates to accommodate their conflicting responses to women defendants was one of targeting women into two groups – those who it could be agreed merited compassion and those who did not. The binary stereotyping of women defendants is well documented but its strategic value to magistrates has been less well examined. In order to act, despite the contradictions in their practices, magistrates draw on their own life experience to decide whether or not they can define or recognize the conditions which appear to explain or excuse women's criminal activity. The key components in this targeting process are a) the extent of woman's domestic responsibilities, b) the extent to which her appearance, demeanour, and life-style accord with sexual 'normality', and c) the extent to which her problems can be pathologized and 'treated'. In short, the woman defendant is constructed within the discourses of *domesticity, sexuality,* and *pathology.*

Domesticity

Women are treated no differently from men, except where
there are domestic circumstances – that's only natural.

(Magistrate 2 – female)

Two different arguments were propounded for the consideration by magistrates of women's domestic responsibilities, although these were frequently conflated. First, domestic problems were seen to explain or excuse female crime (which, of itself, was assumed to be unnatural). Women might be reduced to breaking the law either directly by insufferable husbands ('Women aren't naturally criminal – it's the men that force them into it'), or indirectly by the pressures of family life:

A married woman, and especially a mother, is the keystone of
the family and is subject to great strains and tensions,
particularly if in a 'one-parent family' situation or when the
husband is unemployed. This could push a woman into crime,
particularly, in my opinion, shoplifting or attempting to obtain
benefits to which she would not be entitled.

(Magistrate 8 – female)

Domestic problems may also lead to alcohol abuse which, in turn, was recognized as an explanation of crime – provided either that treatment was being sought (and the problem could thus be pathologized) or that the shaky hand was still rocking the cradle (cf. Curlee 1968 in Otto 1981).

A woman stabbed her husband in a pub recently – we were
lenient because she was going to have treatment for her
alcohol problem.

(Magistrate 6 – male)

Alcoholism is increasing in women. We dealt with a woman
who was drunk in charge of a child in a pub. I thought – it's
better than leaving the baby at home!

(Magistrate 4 – female)

Second, domestic responsibilities were also important in the
mitigation of sentence. The effect of a sentence on a woman's
family was often considered more important than the effect on
the woman herself. Imprisoning women with children was agreed
to be a very last resort, primarily because of the consequences for
the children:

Trying and sentencing a mother has its problems for me
because I look at her situation, taking into account the effect
upon her family.

(Magistrate 7 – female)

In cases where women have in their care babies or young
children I feel that magistrates explore every possible sentence
other than imprisonment.

(Magistrate 8 – female)

Despite this, there are some 1600 children with mothers in prison
(NACRO 1986) and that is not, perhaps, surprising when one
considers the irony of this remark from one woman magistrate:

The governor at one women's prison told me once, 'Women
should come here for at least six months, then we can train
them to be good mothers and they're grateful'.

Motherhood, *per se*, does not protect women from imprisonment
and magistrates do not take kindly to women whom they perceive
to be 'blackmailing' them with their domestic responsibilities
(Walker 1985). The issue in question is whether or not the
defendant is a *good* mother, that is, conforming to conventional,
middle-class expectations of appropriate motherhood and

wifeliness (Edwards 1985). Mothers who commit crimes are, almost by definition, bad mothers who need training to be good mothers. Ironically, such training may require their removal from the site of mothering to a site of punishment. In order, on the one hand, to disrupt the sequence of mothering minimally, 'punishment' should be kept to a minimum. On the other hand, to improve the technical quality of mothering, 'training' needs to be extensive. Pat Carlen (1983) discovered that these ironies are not lost on those women who experience them and that their typical response was not one of conspicuous gratitude.

Sexuality

A woman in charge of an office who cooks the books gets no sympathy from me – I treat her like a man.

(Magistrate 9 – male)

The corollary of marking positively (Ardener 1978) women defendants with domestic responsibilities is marking negatively those without them. Within this latter category, two groups appeared to receive little sympathy from magistrates. Young single women who committed offences in company posed a threat to conventional images of femininity and challenged magistrates' authority:

They don't give reasons – just shrug their shoulders.

(Magistrate 2 – female)

Such 'dumb insolence' was not expected from women defendants since it did not accord with stereotypical expectations of women as guilt-ridden and anxious to please. Defiance manifested in dress, posture, or speech is typically a masculine attribute and women who displayed such an attitude risked alienating magistrates whose personal life experience did not equip them to 'identify with' such a lack of femininity.

Similarly, older women in positions of authority in their work were unlikely to be viewed as meriting compassion. Like women magistrates, they had entered a public world dominated by men. While their aggressiveness and competitiveness were seen as more legitimate than the defiance of younger defendants, the price they had to pay for breaking the law was that of being treated (by implication more harshly) 'like a man'.

Criminal activity that could not be attributed to domestic responsibility tended to be viewed as an expression of sexuality or, more specifically, a lack of femininity. Certain crimes were identified as 'women's' crimes. Shoplifting, soliciting, Social Security fraud, and embezzlement could be recognized as gender-role expressive (Edwards 1985). Other crimes were less acceptable:

> I think that perhaps, in the past, women did receive more sympathy from courts than men, but with the increasing number of women appearing for various crimes, particularly those usually committed by men, I think their attitude is changing.
>
> (Magistrate 8 – female)

As Heidensohn (1985: 94) observes, 'offences which have apparently nothing to do with sexuality are – when committed by women – transformed into expressions of female sexuality or the lack of it'.

Pathology

> We ask for reports more often on women – they often have problems of 'change of life' or medication.
>
> (Magistrate 6 – male)

Closely associated with the image of women defendants as 'sexual' is a further assumption that they are 'sick'. As we have seen, magistrates are fairly sceptical about psychiatric diagnoses and, consequently, those I interviewed did not feel they had come across much 'proper' mental illness among women defendants. Nevertheless, the ascription of what might be described as 'sub-psychiatric' medical conditions to women defendants was widespread.

In the construction of femininity, the 'normal' female body and mind are perceived as being predisposed to malfunction. Menstruation, pregnancy, childbirth, and the menopause all result in 'hormonal imbalance' – a phrase which connotes that women may themselves be 'imbalanced' during those times. This principle of 'periodicity' (Luckhaus 1985) implies that there are times when the mood and behaviour of even the 'normal' woman is likely to be so adversely affected by her biology that any subsequent criminal activity may be regarded as at least partially consequent on it and excused by it. The dilemma posed for lay magistrates is that of assessing the eligibility of a woman defendant for inclusion in this 'excused' category. Is this particular woman 'genuinely' unbalanced and disturbed or is she a malingerer? Because of the 'periodic' nature of her alleged disturbance, it is quite possible for any woman to appear 'normal' in court while claiming that she was 'abnormal' at the time of her offence. To resolve this socio-legal conundrum magistrates have to rely on information supplied by 'experts' in medical and social inquiry reports. But magistrates reserve the right to use their common sense to evaluate the information provided by experts and even when the expert has a relatively undisputed 'authority to know' – as a psychiatrist undoubtedly does – his claims may still be weak because common sense denies any need for that particular area of knowing (Huntington 1981). Information from general practitioners and probation officers was generally accorded more respect by magistrates than that from psychiatrists:

> Older women give medical reasons, produce a doctor's certificate. We have to take that into account because doctors don't write those lightly.
>
> (Magistrate 2 – female)

> I think we pay more attention to what the probation officer says than the psychiatrist – *they* seem to state the obvious.
>
> (Magistrate 1 – female)

The discourse of pathology reinforces beliefs about the natural contrariness of women and about women being 'at the mercy of their raging hormones' (Luckhaus 1985).

Implications for sentencing

Although magistrates believed that they tried hard not to send women to prison, they were not enthusiastic advocates of alternative disposals. Domestic responsibilities were seen to preclude most women defendants from doing Community Service and one magistrate expressed a novel variation on that theme:

> Community Service is usually done in someone's spare time – women don't have any!
>
> (Magistrate 6 – male)

This comment could be seen as reinforcing a view expressed to me by a probation officer responsible for selecting candidates for Community Service, that a woman might be rejected where it was felt that her husband would object to her being out of the home on a Sunday and thus impose additional domestic pressure on her. Alternatively, it could be seen as reflecting a deeper concern about the justice of requiring society's largest group of unpaid workers to perform even more 'voluntary' work as punishment (Dominelli 1984). Women's lack of financial competence also embarrassed magistrates (Carlen 1983) and presented difficulties in the imposition of fines. The absence of an independent income frequently meant that a woman's fine would have to be paid by her husband, although some magistrates felt this to be no bad thing, especially in the case of television licence offences.[1]

> In some cases it should be the husbands in court – when it's TV licence or leaving the wife without money.
>
> (Magistrate 10 – male)

Unsurprisingly, the sentence most favoured by magistrates for women was the probation order, since this offered the least disruption to a woman's domestic situation and enabled her problems to be individualized and pathologized. Probation was invariably advocated on 'welfare' grounds (Eaton 1985) and little consideration seemed to be given to the implications of such a sentence for a woman's position on the sentencing 'tariff'. Recent attempts by the Probation Service to raise the tariff weighting of probation orders and render them credible as direct alternatives to custody for more serious offenders (Home Office 1984) were implicitly regarded as irrelevant to women, who were assumed to be characteristically 'one-off' offenders rather than recidivists (Pearson 1976). The consequence for women who do reoffend, however, may be to escalate their progress up an already truncated tariff[2] towards a custodial sentence, regardless of the severity (or lack of severity) of their offences.

Together, the discourses of domesticity, sexuality, and pathology provide a complex of excusing and mitigating explanations of female crime which was accepted fairly uncritically by the male magistrates I interviewed. The women magistrates, however, appeared to experience a much greater degree of ambivalence and discomfort in relation to women defendants and this was recognized by one or two of their more perceptive male colleagues:

> Women offenders are different physically and emotionally – more complex. I don't understand them as well as women magistrates do. But women magistrates are sometimes harder – perhaps they feel that women who offend have let the side down.

(Magistrate 6 – male)

SISTERS IN LAW? WOMEN JUDGING WOMEN

Women magistrates are socially constructed within a number of discourses, in such a way that they can claim to be both similar to (for the purposes of special and authoritative understanding) and different from (for the purposes of sentencing) women defendants. They may be located within two definitional sites. First, as women in positions of authority over other women, they may be regarded as 'wise women' (Heidensohn 1985: 167). Alongside women prison officers, women nurses, and women social workers (including women probation officers), they stand between the demands of the patriarchal state and the mass of women on whom those demands are made, translating 'expert knowledge' into 'common sense' for the consumption of the always and already failing women (Hutter and Williams 1981). Second, as magistrates they are part of the complex machinery of control (Carlen 1976), which characterizes 'amateur justice' (Burney 1979). The deconstruction of the 'women judging women' complex therefore involves the excavation of a number of layers of social relations. The foundation of the relationship lies deeper than moral outrage consequent on a sense of womanhood betrayed[3] and spotlights the interplay of class and gender issues in the court-room.

Images of women magistrates

We're told that we're representing the Queen, and I think
some of them feel they need to look like her!

(Magistrate 11 – female)

None of us women magistrates wear hats – we're unique, I
think! I won't wear one. I get confused in a hat. My head gets
hot and I get hopeless.

(Mrs Christian Annersley, in Blythe 1969: 251)

It is not difficult to conjure up a mental picture of a 'typical' woman
magistrate (cf. Pearson 1976). She is white, middle-aged to elderly,
middle- or upper-class, the wife of a local dignitary or a retired
headmistress. She may or may not have children of her own but she
knows how they should be reared. She will invariably have 'done
good' and wear a hat. Yet, as Mrs Annersley's account of her work
indicates, this was not a totally accurate picture even twenty years
ago. While the women I interviewed could all be described as
'typical' in their age, class, and background, they were neither rigid
nor ignorant in their opinions and gave the impression of wanting
to understand crime and women criminals in particular. They
recognized that their personal life experience was privileged, in the
socio-economic sense of the word, and that this sometimes
restricted the usefulness of 'privileging' that experience in the sense
of using it to inform their judgements. They were certainly not
incapable of sympathizing and identifying with the problems
experienced by the women defendants as 'not like us' because the
consequences of any alternative interpretation were too painful to
contemplate. Those consequences would threaten the all-
important notion of consensus to which magisterial common sense
is committed. Over-identification by women magistrates with the
oppression of women defendants might oblige women magistrates
to challenge the dominance of their male colleagues on the Bench.
So while a woman magistrate may be recruited to ensure a 'balance
of the sexes', she is prohibited by the imperative of consensus from
fully expressing her 'femaleness' in her practice on the Bench. The
'knowledge' about women defendants which she is authorized to
have by reason of her own status as a *woman* magistrate is rendered

inferior and inappropriate by reason of her subordination to male magistrates. If 'real' criminals are men, then 'real' magistrates are also men, and the women who invade the public space of the court-room in positions of power and authority are expected to emulate the qualities of reason, 'objectivity' – and sexism – demonstrated by their male colleagues.

What then are the conditions which determine relationships which women magistrates have a) with their colleagues and b) with women defendants?

Achieving consensus and the simultaneous recognition and denial of difference

We think of ourselves as a nice team.

(Mrs Christian Annersley)

Lay magistrates are selected both for their differences and for their ability to 'get on' with each other. They are, in theory at least, expected to demonstrate that they are 'moderate, fair and conscientious: decent people picked for their ability to get on with other decent people' (Burney 1979: 212). Yet, precisely because magistrates are encouraged to rely on their own experiences and senses, the scope for conflict between them would, at first sight, appear to be considerable. An outsider might question the extent of material and ideological difference existing between magistrates (Baldwin and Bottomley 1978; Hood 1962) but there is a high level of 'felt' or perceived difference among magistrates themselves.

We get a wide spread of occupations on our Bench.

(Magistrate 1 – female)

Yet though this view was endorsed by most magistrates I interviewed they all put emphasis upon the relative ease with which consensus was achieved, despite these differences. Differ-ence was recognized but only to be cast aside.

I venture to suggest that this is one of the strengths of the Bench – that it is comprised of men and women of different opinions who eventually make a *unanimous* decision.

(Magistrate 12 – female)

> We usually all agree. I've not been in a situation of real conflict.
>
> (Magistrate 8 – female)

The point here is that, while magistrates normally sit in threes – a system designed to accommodate the expression of differing opinions – they routinely experience the system as one of agreement or consensus. This is particularly significant for women magistrates who feel prohibited from even expressing certain of their instinctive responses because they may be 'too personal' and 'too individualized' to be acceptable to their male colleagues. Such inhibition led one woman magistrate to protest (too loudly?):

> We have a wonderful relationship on our Bench – we don't mind whom we sit with. There's no difference between men and women on the Bench – the women can be *just as fierce.*
>
> (Magistrate 2 – emphasis added)

Thus, women magistrates who can sublimate or deny their womanhood are celebrated, for magisterial common sense; the guardian of public morality can thus claim to be gender-neutral in practice and in law. But gender-neutrality is a myth and the imperative of consensus ultimately robs magisterial common sense of the power that might result from genuine gender conflicts. The guardians of public morality are either men, or those women who will accept a male-defined consensus. The only personal life experience which is, in reality, given special status or authority in the court-room is that of male magistrates. It is not then surprising that women magistrates exercise caution in their judgements of women defendants.

Women defendants: like-us-yet-not-like-us

While the male magistrates I interviewed were relatively content to attribute female crime to domestic strains and responsibilities, the women magistrates tended to expect women either to accept their lot and make the best of it, or to be more 'rational' and discriminating in the remedies they sought. There was no lack of understanding of the difficulties:

> I was on a baby-battering case. With all my children, I know what a strain it must be without a supportive husband....
>
> (Magistrate 4)

but these were not accepted as excusing conditions. Another woman magistrate echoed the sentiment:

> I can understand a young mother without a supportive husband getting desperate – but not hitting little babies. Why don't they take it out on their husbands?

> (Magistrate 3)

Why indeed? One may well ask. The dilemma for these magistrates was that their own experiences, on which they were relying, did not equip them fully to understand the woman defendant because *common* sense does not allow for different material circumstances. Yet they felt unable to go beyond that experience to recognize the validity of generalizable statements about power relations within the family. Magisterial common sense requires that the unspoken common condition of this contradiction (namely, power relations) be excluded, or at least only partially expressed. Thus, in the last instance quoted the magistrate recognizes the power relation between mother and child while refusing to acknowledge the effectivity of that between husband and wife.

Even more ambivalence was expressed by women magistrates about the attribution of the criminal activity of women to their biology. In this, they were not expressing concern about the dangers for all women of the medicalization of women's behaviour, nor were they arguing that such reductionism:

> impugns the integrity of the female actor, stripping her action of cultural and political meaning and anaesthetising the social and economic origin and conditions in which that action takes place.

> (Luckhaus 1985: 177)

Rather, such conditions were excluded because the magistrates had not – or claimed to have not – experienced such conditions for themselves:

> Menopause is used frequently as a defence – I'm not very sympathetic. I tell my male colleagues, I'll let them know what really happens *when it happens to me*....Pre-menstrual tension – *my girls* don't seem to suffer....

> (Magistrate 4 – emphases added)

As a woman and mother of three grown-up daughters, I believe
that women have to recognize and accept any variations in
their behaviour due to the menstrual cycle, and not use this as
an excuse.

(Magistrate 12)

The ability of women defendants to touch very primitive
emotions of sadness and sympathy in women magistrates is a
taboo subject. It is something not to be shared and examined but
to be hidden away and denied because it is too threatening to the
dominant ideologies about crime, justice, and masculinity.

Discussion about women defendants was thus foreclosed by
women magistrates with the symbolic phrase, 'I can understand
but...'. The shared condition of female experience was recognized
but such a recognition represented the challenge of the Other –
the disruptive intrusion of an alternative, non-legitimated mode
of lived experience. Such a challenge must be confronted and
controlled. So the moment of recognition passes and the space
for negotiation opened up by the challenge is re-closed.

The women magistrates I spoke to were not the female
equivalents of 'Disgusted, Tunbridge Wells'. They were women
who felt confused about the extent to which they could claim to
understand other women. They were women who often did
understand, but who did not trust their own understanding. They
seemed to feel acutely that they were living in a man's world and
that they must locate themselves in a symbolic universe of
meanings that were empirically grounded in male, rather than
female experience.

CONCLUSION

The relationship between magistrates and defendants is
constructed within a discourse of common sense which, despite
its inherent paradoxes and discontinuities, is represented as a
consistent and coherent unity. Although magisterial common
sense may appear to challenge and transgress 'expert' discourse, it
is in fact a competing discourse of 'expertise'. In relation to
women defendants, it is characterized by a three-fold myth:

1) That magistrates are disqualified from knowing anything
about women defendants because knowledge accrues through

experience and, since women defendants are always and already invisible, they are inaccessible to the senses and therefore unknowable (yet forever known).

2) That magistrates can never generalize about women defendants *qua* women, because the law is blind to differences of gender (as of class, age, race, etc.); they treat every case 'on its merit' and see women defendants as intractably heterogeneous.

3) That magistrates can always reach a consensus about women defendants both because of and despite the social, economic, political, or, specifically, gender differences of their personal life experiences, these differences being hailed (at the point of recruitment to the Bench) and denied (at the point of judgment) in the interests of justice.

These judicial myths have been challenged and it has been argued that:

1) Magistrates act 'as though' they have knowledge of women defendants, that knowledge emanating from cultural stereotypes of appropriate female behaviour and being reinforced by their own socially and discursively privileged personal life experience.

2) Magistrates invoke the ostensibly gender-neutral moral concept of merit to justify treating women defendants *qua* women differently from male defendants, since meritorious conduct in men and women is differentially defined.

3) Women magistrates suppress their empathetic under-standing of women's position in society because, having entered the masculine world of the criminal justice system by virtue of their womanhood, their ability to sustain their authority and credibility within it is dependent on their denial of that womanhood. The judging of women by women magistrates is seen to be doubly authoritative because women magistrates can root their claim to an authoritative understanding of female law-breakers in the paradoxical claim that (with female law-breakers) they themselves share a biological experience common to all women without using it as an excuse to break the law.

Nevertheless, the analyses of this chapter suggest that a greater understanding of women defendants by the magistracy might be achieved if women magistrates felt more confident – and were allowed – to express their genuinely differing perspectives and opinions. The structure for such a richness and variety of contribution exists; what is lacking is the will to experience the discomfort of conflict, especially when the mechanism for achieving an apparent consensus – the appeal to and of common sense – is so readily available. Women magistrates, like women defendants, are socially constructed within the discourses of domesticity, sexuality, and pathology. The evidence of this chapter suggests that though women magistrates and women defendants may indeed be 'sisters in law', subject to a common gender oppression, they are not yet able fully to recognize each other because of a) their class differences; and b) the judicial ideology that claims that law is both class- and gender-neutral.

Chapter Five

GUILTY WOMEN?

The construction of female law-breakers within the discourses of domesticity, sexuality, and pathology by judicial, medical, and welfare personnel is a unifying theme of this study, but one of the unique contributions of solicitors to this construction is their authorization, within legal and judicial discourse, to recognize the guilty mind. The term 'recognize' is not used here to imply any positivistic imperative to search out 'the truth'. On the contrary, the ideology of legal representation releases the solicitor from any such moral obligation. The relationship between solicitors and their clients (whether male or female) is determined by the legal condition that solicitors must suspend any inclination to disbelieve what their clients say. Legal representation is constructed as being morally neutral; lawyers are engaged for their technical expertise – for their knowledge of the law and their ability to articulate the application of its principles to a particular case. Their desire to obtain a favourable outcome for their clients stems from professional disinterest and not from any personal commitment to, or even belief in, the client's reading of events. 'Recognition' here refers to the process whereby solicitors construct a coherent unity (viz. *mens rea*) out of the contradictions that surface from efforts to address the Other of legal discourse, namely, the organization of the difference that constitutes the 'guilt/innocence' distinction.

The distinctive nature of the organization of that difference in relation to women is that women are both ideologically and materially preconditioned to accept the description of 'guilty'. Ideologically, many women experience a generalized sense of (moral) guilt consequent on their perception of themselves as failed wives and mothers, a perception which emanates from discourses which construct women as always and already lacking (Carlen and Worrall 1987). This all-pervading sense of guilt predisposes some women to accept readily that certain of their specific actions can/should be described as 'guilty' acts which, by implication, require punishment. Pauline provided an example of such reasoning:

> I expected a lot worse and, quite honestly, I felt I deserved a lot worse – I still do. I've said this to Dr C many times – I still feel that I haven't been punished. At the back of my mind I feel, 'I've got off very lightly'.

The ideological conditions which predispose some women towards an admission of legal guilt are reinforced by the material conditions surrounding their appearance in court. A decision to plead guilty may be influenced by any or all of the following material considerations:

1) inability to resist police questioning (Dell 1971);

2) likelihood of being remanded in custody if a 'not guilty' plea is entered (Home Office 1983; NACRO 1983) and the consequences for any children;

3) likelihood of being a 'first offender' and therefore ignorant of procedures and rights;

4) the particular difficulty of prostitutes proving their innocence where it is only their word against that of the police (McLeod 1982);

5) the sheer lack of 'guts to stand up in court and put her case' (Dell 1971);

6) the desire to 'get it over with' in order to avoid the feared stigma of publicity which might damage relationships with family and neighbours.

Thus, immediate concerns about the delays and adjournments which inevitably result from entering pleas of 'not guilty' may outweigh any consideration of possible future discrimination consequent on acquiring a criminal record. Suzanne Dell (1971) argued that access to legal representation appeared to reduce the tendency to plead inconsistently (that is, to plead guilty when one believes oneself to be innocent). The evidence from my interviews with solicitors did not support this optimism. On the contrary, most of the male solicitors seemed more ready to agree with Pollak (1950) that women's criminality was more likely to be masked by their innate deviousness than to be unjustly or inappropriately attributed to them:

> It's sometimes difficult to convince women that they are in the wrong. They say 'I forgot' and sometimes plead 'not guilty', but they're always found 'guilty'.
>
> (Solicitor 1)

> I have the impression that quite a high proportion of the embezzlement type of offence (cooking the books) is committed by women and it is exceptionally hard to convince them that they are in fact guilty.
>
> (Solicitor 2)

> I doubt if there are many first offender shoplifters – only first time caught.
>
> (Solicitor 3)

Implicit in these remarks is the assumption, outlined above, that the 'normal' woman pleads guilty because she feels guilty (and it is unnecessary to clarify whether that sense of guilt is general to being a woman or specific to the behaviour in question). It may also be related to the irrational assumption that because most normal women do not appear in court on criminal charges those who do must be real criminals – that is, they must have committed not only this crime but several more before. Consequently, the woman who denies guilt is abnormal. Ironically, however, the woman who appears too ready to admit guilt – and lacks the more general sense of moral guilt – is also deemed abnormal:

> Female crime is less hidden nowadays – women are less ashamed to admit to it – they are more liberated.
>
> (Solicitor 3)

Given this apparent presumption of guilt, it is not perhaps surprising that some of the women in this study were sceptical of the value of representation. Carol was unhappy about her solicitor's reluctance to defend her (as opposed to mitigating for her) and Ivy preferred to try and defend herself. Maureen blamed herself for being unable to give her solicitor enough evidence for a defence. Underlying these accounts was a common concern among the women that they were unable to communicate what they really wanted to say in a way that would be listened to, heard, and recognized by their (predominantly male) solicitors. The prospect of attempting to justify one's actions (indeed, one's existence) to a man whose education and background may be such as to place him well beyond the class of person with whom the woman would normally have any social dealings whatsoever, let alone of any intimate nature, may be simply too daunting to contemplate.

Finally, and more prosaically, women may be discouraged from engaging a solicitor because of the expense. The cost of legal representation may appear prohibitive to a woman who, though without income herself, may be married to a man whose income excludes him from receiving free Legal Aid. It may be a particularly daunting prospect if such cost is likely to fall on a husband whose response to her predicament is not conspicuously supportive.

'WOMEN OFFENDERS ARE NEEDY, GREEDY, OR SICK'

Just as magistrates tended to disqualify themselves as competent speakers about female law-breakers on the grounds that such women are 'invisible' by reason of their numerical insignificance and that magistrates are therefore inevitably 'inexperienced' in dealing with them, so a number of solicitors initially minimized the difference in courts' (and, by implication, their own) treatment of male and female law-breakers.

> I would say there is no difference between the sexes so far as verdict is concerned. I cannot think that there is any other difference in this connection and, for example, I do not feel that a woman would be fined either more or less heavily. The difference is only noticeable over the question of deprivation of liberty.
>
> (Solicitor 4)

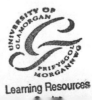

From a prosecution point of view I cannot see that there are any particular problems associated with prosecuting women. From a defence point of view I think that the only problem which does arise occasionally is in connection with the 'menopausal shoplifter' who may find giving instructions to a male solicitor embarrassing.

(Solicitor 5)

I find no difference between men and women in taking instructions except where 'sensitive' mitigation is involved – for example, menopause or pregnancy.

(Solicitor 1)

On further enquiry, however, it became apparent that the process of 'normalizing' female law-breakers involved solicitors in defining or describing them as being located within a restricted number of gender-specific categories in relation to a) the nature of their offences, b) their motivational explanations, and c) their appropriate treatment.

The nature of their offences

The normalization process begins with the recognition of the offence and there is evidence that solicitors see female law-breakers primarily as shoplifters and, to a lesser extent, as fraudsters.

So many of the shoplifting cases involve women and follow the same pattern (middle-aged, on nerve tablets, mind on other things, no previous convictions). One is left with the feeling that although most are quite properly convicted of theft it is somehow a 'different' offence. They would never remotely consider any other form of dishonesty – and yet steal from a shop.

(Solicitor 2)

You quite regularly come across them in shoplifting cases because women don't commit that many other kinds of crime – you don't get many women burglars or many who are involved in violence – it's mainly theft, quite a lot of social security frauds.

(Solicitor 6)

Such observations would seem to be confirmed by the official criminal statistics (Box 1983: 166). Shoplifting is the only offence which is apparently committed by equal numbers of men and women but the explanation for this is by no means self-evident. The presence of women in shops and, to a lesser extent, social security offices is far more 'congruous' than at the scene of burglaries or public brawls (Worrall 1981). Surveillance of women, therefore, tends to focus on the former locations and if women do indeed have their 'minds on other things', they may be careless enough to make their theft obvious to skilled observers. (Alternatively, having their 'mind on other things' could be interpreted as negating any intent to steal and therein lies a significant dilemma for solicitors.)

In less congruous locations, however, a certain expeditious 'blindness' seems to afflict witnesses and the police. Even when women burglars and muggers *are* 'seen', the assumption remains that, if they are accompanied by men, they cannot be as dangerous as their male companions:

> Women's different treatment starts before court. The police don't prosecute women in joint offences if the men plead guilty. They want to get the women home – for example, in cases of receiving stolen goods.
>
> (Solicitor 4)

> Women have been involved with men in burglaries and the police haven't bothered to prosecute the women. I can't give you names, of course, but it definitely happens. They only want the men.
>
> (Solicitor 7)

The rightful place for 'normal' women is in the home and the myth persists that women don't (or can't) burgle. But the Pollak myth of masked female criminality is discredited when women on their own are seen committing serious offences and these may consequently be over-reported (Hindelang 1979) because of the 'incongruity' between their actions and the 'normal' behaviour of women. One arena where the violent woman is taken very seriously is the domestic:

> If you have a wife who beats her husband, that's a very

extraordinary state of affairs, and is looked on as the exception rather than the rule. I prosecuted one not very long ago where the woman had stabbed her husband and obviously the first thing you look at is psychiatric problems.

(Solicitor 6)

Women who use weapons to assault their husbands or boy-friends are often depicted in court as engaging in cold-blooded and pre-meditated action (Dobash and Dobash 1979; Edwards 1984). To counteract such images, and thus to 'render them harmless' (Allen 1987a), solicitors have to redefine motivation, as in the example given, in terms of 'psychiatric problems'. Yet the women themselves often see their action as self-defence or perhaps, more accurately, as self-preservation (for, in law, self-defence must be a response to an immediate threat of harm, whereas assaults on husbands or boy-friends may be the result of cumulative threats or assaults over a period of time and thus, strictly speaking, lack the requisite element of spontaneity). As Carlen found, 'They justified their own extreme acts of violence on the grounds that legitimate and effective protest was not open to women' (1983: 42). Had women learned (or had they the physical strength for) the more culturally acceptable forms of violence, such as punching, kicking, and wrestling, they might not have resorted to more extreme and lethal forms of assault.

Another blow to the myth of masked female criminality is struck by those unchivalrous men who are themselves under threat of imprisonment:

AW: Do you ever feel that women are actually taking the blame for offences that have been committed by men?

Solicitor: I have known situations where the husband is on a suspended sentence and it's the meter – that's the classic. It does happen, yes. But, by and large, it's only cases in the domestic environment that you can do that – not in a burglary, if he's caught redhanded. If you're both in the supermarket, you can take the whole blame and say he didn't know, when he probably did – or the DHSS cheque that's forged....

Their motivational explanations

The acceptable (and thus recognizable) motivational explanations of female crime both differ from and are more rigidly categorized than those of male crime. Solicitor 8 put it succinctly:

Women offenders are needy, greedy, or sick!

Explanations of 'need', 'greed', and 'sickness' are 'offender-specific', in the sense that they are rooted in the personality and pathology of the individual offender. By contrast, explanations of male crime have become increasingly 'offence-' and 'situation-specific' (e.g., McGuire and Priestley 1985), thus testifying both to the greater social acceptability of male crime and the greater willingness of courts to consider a variety of motivational accounts in the cases of male law-breakers.

Ironically, however, although such 'offender-specific' explanations appear to be concerned with the uniqueness of each offender, their homely familiarity absolves both speaker and listener from the obligation to investigate further the account of any individual woman law-breaker. It is already assumed that all accounts will ultimately fit into one of these categories, from which can be automatically deduced the 'correct' response. Not only is it assumed that all accounts *will* ultimately fit, but it is also assumed that there is no disagreement about the criteria for categorization. Solicitors and magistrates have no difficulty in 'knowing' in which category to place a particular account – even though there may seem to be times when solicitors may feel they ought to challenge such assumed 'knowledge':

It isn't really a doctor they need – it's a cheque book.

(Solicitor 6)

The implication of such a challenge would be that the boundaries between the 'needy', the 'greedy', and the 'sick' are not as clear and self-evident as one might like to believe. But the utterance of such a challenge contains within it its own source of remedy and absolution, for it allows the recognition of an economic explanation of crime, while simultaneously absolving both speaker and listener of the consequences of such recognition. It may be obvious that it is a cheque book which is needed but it is equally obvious that neither the speaker nor the listener is in a position to provide it and the solicitor will only irritate the magistrate by suggesting otherwise. The recognition of 'a cheque book need' is extra-judicial. It is not an excusing condition and must therefore be represented as 'a doctor need'. Thus, solicitors discover that the redefinition of need as sickness serves to ease both their own and magistrates' discomfort. But the effectiveness of such redefinition is also dependent on the perceived severity of the illegal action. The more serious an offence is perceived to be, the more likely it is that its motivation will be accounted for in terms of 'sickness', provided the nature of the offence remains compatible with the essential 'nature' of woman-hood. If, however, the crime is perceived to be both serious and 'unnatural', its motivation may well be accounted for in terms of inherent wickedness or 'greed'. But the motivational rationale of 'greed' is not only employed in relation to 'serious, unnatural' offences. A petty offence (such as the stolen Yorkie bar cited below) may not be considered worthy of categorization as a symptom of either 'need' or 'sickness'. It may be considered worthy only of contempt and thus fall, by default, into the category of 'greed'. This particular example also demonstrates the power of the vocabulary of food in relation to women. A Yorkie bar is self-evidently not a neces-sity. It is an un-needed luxury, the motivation for whose acquisition can only be rendered understandable in terms of 'greed', with its implication of 'self-indulgence' and 'selfishness' – an implication which is anathema to the acceptable image of women as 'selfless' and 'self-sacrificing'. Greed, therefore, need not be demonstrated only in serious offences – larger-scale thefts or frauds. Greed is the category into which all motivational accounts fall that cannot be recognized in alternative terms. Greed is the category which invokes contempt rather than sympathy and justifies punishment rather than treat-ment. It is the category which releases the speaker and the listener from any inordinate struggle for justice, for it is assumed that no response to greed can be inherently unjust – all that has to be de-cided is the classical consideration of proportion. Justice in response to greed is thus transformed from a qualitative to a quantitative issue.

Their appropriate treatment

In the light of these restrictions on the categories of offence and motivation within which female law-breakers could be 'appropriately' located by solicitors, it is not perhaps surprising that they should also be seen as requiring gender-congruent treatment – that is, treatment which attends to their 'sickness' or 'neediness'.

The solicitors I spoke to expressed considerable ambivalence about the use of strictly 'medical' mitigation in relation to women. They recognized its benefits (as they saw them) but they were also conscious that its reception by magistrates could be miscalculated and their own credibility damaged as a result. But they expressed no such reservations about what might be described as a 'sub-medical' mitigation, with its emphasis on individual 'neediness' (and inadequacy). Such mitigations frequently result in the making of probation orders:

> Women are proportionately more likely to be placed on probation than men; in 1982 they made up 12 per cent of those sentenced by the courts, but 30 per cent of those placed on probation.

> (Walker and Beaumont 1985: 69)

But, as Walker argues, this does not necessarily indicate leniency. It is true that Community Service is rarely used for women (5 per cent of all such orders made in 1982 were on women – Home Office 1983) and most solicitors saw it (or said that magistrates would see it) as an inappropriate disposal for women. Equally, solicitors were reluctant to recommend fines, because they often did recognize the reality of many women offenders' poverty. The probation order, therefore, was the disposal most favoured by solicitors and this appeared to be so for two reasons. First, in the event of the women's exclusion from the 'socially exculpatory' and 'legally effective' (Edwards 1984) category of 'sickness', the probation order provided an alternative route whereby responsibility for her actions could be removed from the woman. Second, the probation order would provide an appropriate arena in which the woman could be encouraged to talk. (The implication here was that the appropriate arena was the private domain of the home, rather than the public domain of the court-room, where it was considered inappropriate for women to talk.)

> I wouldn't put responsibility for the offending on her mental make-up at all. I think to shove it on to psychiatry is taking the back door. I would much sooner shove it on to probation,

because I think the anxiety can be alleviated just as well by sitting and talking, as by taking half a dozen pills every day.

(Solicitor 6)

By recommending probation orders, solicitors thus exhorted women to talk in private for the purposes of transforming themselves into 'normal' women but not to talk in public for the purposes of justifying themselves or challenging the stereotyping of women. Thus the process of normalizing female law-breakers through solicitors' discourse rendered them muted.

THE STAGING OF WOMEN'S RE-PRESENTATION WITHIN THE DISCOURSES OF DOMESTICITY, SEXUALITY, AND PATHOLOGY

Since the majority of people processed through the courts are from the working classes (Box 1983), it is perhaps unsurprising that defendants (both men and women) are encouraged to view their own speech as inferior and in need of translation in order to be understood. As Bernstein (1971, quoted in Carlen 1976) has argued, their restricted linguistic code serves to reinforce only the *form* of the social relationship in which they find themselves. 'Access to an elaborated code will depend on access to specialised social positions within the social structure' (Bernstein 1971, quoted in Carlen 1976: 103). In the court-room, elaborated code is made available only to the experts.

Women are further subordinated, partly because they are already subject to the ideological pressures of gender-role stereotyping outside the court and partly because of the arguably 'masculine' characteristics of the court-room. First, the public nature of the court-room and its communications, reflecting distinctions between 'male' (public) and 'female' (private) space, may seem especially oppressive to women. Second, the adversarial nature of English court proceedings (with their accompanying vocabulary of 'fighting', 'winning', and 'losing') may be seen as irrelevantly aggressive by women. Hence, the expectation of women defendants is not merely that what they say about themselves requires translation, but that they do not have anything to say about themselves. This is perhaps hardly surprising. Since women are seen as 'behaving' rather than 'acting' when they break the law, and since they are seen to be incapable of thinking and making decisions, it is reasonable to assume that they need to be explained, rather than to explain. (The fact that more trouble is not taken to ensure that women are represented, however, suggests that courts are not really very interested in listening to any explanations, preferring rather the comfort of unchallenged assumptions.)

The task of the solicitor in muting the female law-breaker is to construct an acceptable account from those explanations which are 'speakable' and to erase from the record those which are 'unspeakable'. In practice, this involves explaining female law-breakers to the court as normal, feminine women who:

a) ideologically deserve sympathy (the appeal to chivalry) because explanations of their law-breaking are seen to be congruous with 'what are supposed to be their natural, biologically-determined socio-sexual roles and destinies' (Carlen 1985: 10);

b) materially (pragmatically) compel leniency because they can be viewed as 'wives, mothers and sex-objects designed for the satisfaction of male desire' (Carlen 1985: 10).

> I do find that courts are most reluctant to sentence female offenders to terms of imprisonment, particularly when the offender has children and that it is far easier to persuade a court to give a female offender a second or even third chance than it is in the case of male offenders. On reflection, while in some cases this may be as a result of natural sympathy, in other cases it may simply be that the court is recognizing the reality of the situation in that if mother is sent to prison children will have to be taken into Care.
>
> (Solicitor 5)

The reluctance of courts to imprison women, which Solicitor 5 claimed to 'find' (implying a positivistic discovery of the 'truth'), reflected rather the Desire of his own discourse which required him to re-present women within the dominant discourses of femininity – the discourses of domesticity, sexuality, and pathology. But the women in this study constituted a threat to this discourse, since they represented the Other which had to be confronted and controlled.

Domesticity

Solicitors place great emphasis on the construction of female law-breakers as family members, in particular as wives and mothers, with responsibilities that render them deserving of both understanding and sympathy (in relation to the motivation for their offences) and of leniency (in relation to their treatment).

> Courts recognize the importance of the 'competent mother' mitigation. With men it's less important; a magistrate will say, 'I accept that your client is a paragon of virtue – when he is not robbing his employer!'
>
> (Solicitor 8)

> Women often have stronger circumstantial mitigation than men – for example, domestic stress.
>
> (Solicitor 3)

> I use children in mitigation for women but not for men.
>
> (Solicitor 1)

> I think the trappings of being a female offender can sometimes get sympathy, such as having a couple of children who will go into Care if anything happens to you.
>
> (Solicitor 6)

But the 'trappings of being a female offender' do not always or only trap courts into sympathy and leniency. They also provide a trap for the woman herself. As Hilary Walker (1985: 68) argues, courts can sometimes feel that women are trying to blackmail them by 'sheltering' behind their children and can consequently respond in a deliberately punitive way towards the women. There is also increasing evidence that mothers who do not live in nuclear families are less likely to receive sympathy than those who do:

> Judicial misogyny...results in single women, divorced women and women with children in Care [being] more likely to receive custodial sentences than women who, at the time of their court appearances, are living at home with their husbands and children.
>
> (Carlen 1985: 11)

86

It has been further argued (Dominelli 1984: 101) that women are sometimes given less credit for their domestic responsibilities than are those few men with such responsibilities who appear in court (presumably as a result of being 'abandoned' by 'abnormal' women):

> Society's expectation is that women should just 'get on' with their domestic responsibilities and rely on their own resources for doing so.

The trap of domesticity is that at the same time as women are being exhorted to provide for their families many are denied access to legitimate means of provision. By resorting to illegitimate provision they often exclude themselves from the very descriptive category in which they seek, and are exhorted to desire, inclusion:

> CM has a long record, cohabits in overcrowded conditions, has a baby and is pregnant. She was on a suspended sentence. She shoplifted to sell goods for money to pay debts. I thought it was a marvellous thing to do, but the courts had no choice but to send her down.
>
> (Solicitor 7)

Those for whom crime is a rational, if socially unacceptable, response to the conditions of poverty with which society expects them to contend are debarred from articulating such a logic:

> But when they've got no money – well, they often say to you, 'Well, I'll have to do it again' – and where do you go from there? You can't really say that in court. But there's no psychiatry there – it's a deliberate choice – 'I've done it to pay the milkman' – or whatever.
>
> (Solicitor 6)

And therein lies another trap. By offering a rational explanation of her action, which is perceived to be both 'in order' (in so far as it is believed) and 'out of order' (in so far as it is illegitimate), the defendant excludes herself from the possible benefits of psychiatrization.

Finally, the ideal of middle-class domesticity traps a particular class of women whose deprivation itself over-determines their 'suitability' for punishment. Solicitor 4 summarized it thus:

The wife of an estate agent, receiving stolen goods –
respectable, sheltered upbringing, good wife and mother. The
court would think that prison would be so shattering, they'd
keep it to a minimum. Whereas a girl brought up on [a
particularly notorious council estate], knocked about by her
parents and her husband – she'd need a longer sentence to
make any impression!

Respectable, middle-class wives and mothers are assumed to be so
sensitive that they will be reformed by a minimum of punishment
(or no punishment at all). Working-class women are perceived to
be tougher (more like men?) and therefore need to be treated
more harshly if any impression is to be made on them, on the
grounds that punishment is the only thing 'people like that'
understand. Such arguments are reminiscent of medical
discourse in the nineteenth century (Ehrenreich and English
1973) and the politics of the differential treatment of sickness
among middle-class and working-class women. Middle-class
women and those with husbands and children are seen to be
more amenable to non-judicial social controls and less in need of
the controls of the criminal justice system, which are reserved for
those who are without the 'normal' traditional social controls
(the workplace for men; the family for women). Deprivation of
such controls is seen to produce a different 'type' of woman – a
depraved woman who is incapable of making moral choice and is
therefore in need of more direct techniques of behaviour
modification to control her. The 'suitability' of such women for
punishment is, however, reinforced by a contradictory argument
which implies that, despite (or perhaps because of – see Dobash
and Dobash 1979, on the 'appropriate victim') being victims of
abuse, these women *have* made choices. Middle-class magistrates
find it hard to understand the material circumstances which
restrict the choices of such women (for example, the lack of a car
forcing a woman to walk alone at night or the absence of
alternative accommodation forcing a woman to return to a
violent husband). Instead, these women are seen to have chosen
to contribute to their plight by their 'imprudent behaviour'
(Pattullo 1983) and therefore to be at least partially responsible
for its consequences.

Sexuality

Solicitors appear to have fewer inhibitions than other court personnel when it comes to exploiting the overtly sexual impact which female law-breakers may have in court, although this is not an aspect of representation that they would discuss openly with the women themselves. Solicitor 7 demonstrated that 'getting to know the Bench' includes taking account of both the gender and age of magistrates and theorizing about their likely perceptions and expectations of women, based on an understanding of gender power relations within society:

> Courts are very chauvinistic towards women, always softer. If it's a young woman, I think the male magistrates fancy her; if she's older, it's domestic responsibilities. Some of the older women take a moralistic attitude towards prostitutes – 'look what sort of woman she is'. Some of the younger women magistrates are genuinely concerned about young prostitutes – they want to get to the bottom of what makes them do it.

Older men are expected to regard young women primarily as sex objects and the recent increase in awareness of the ideological determinants of incest (or 'father–daughter rape'; Ward 1985) suggests that even the most paternalistic of magistrates cannot escape that reading of his attitudes. In this way, solicitors reinforce the image of the female law-breaker as 'whore', an image which is, as Heidensohn explains (1985: 93), complex and distorting. It is an image which constructs all non-conforming behaviour by women as a reflection of their sexuality.

But there are risks attached to placing too much reliance on this image, for certain expressions of sexuality may threaten to render male magistrates impotent:

> You can get women who cry and cry and that can embarrass men magistrates and upset them and put them off their flow or whatever.

> (Solicitor 6)

If the defendant is an older woman, this fundamental manifestation of power through the construction of women as legitimate objects of sexual desire is overlaid by the ideology of familialism which constructs less attractive or less accessible women as legitimate objects of 'husbandly' respect, pity, and protection – or chastisement (cf. Box 1983). Familialism thus endows male magistrates with the possessive right to maintain such women in powerless and dependent positions by either chivalrous or punitive means. Women magistrates, as we have seen, are faced with the 'like-us-yet-not-like-us' conundrum in dealing with female defendants. Are such women potential sisters and daughters or do they constitute a 'breed apart', whose law-breaking is personally insulting (Dominelli 1984)? Even when female magistrates appear genuine in their concern about young prostitutes, the explanations that seem to assist them in getting 'to the bottom of what makes them do it' are invariably individualistic and frequently pathological.

Pathology

The third ideology that dominated solicitors' discourse in the muting of the female law-breaker was that which allowed her to be re-presented as 'sick'. The extent to which that sickness could be used as a defence negating intent (as opposed to a factor in mitigation) was limited, especially if specifically gynaecological dysfunctions were involved.[1] In a discussion about the relevance of pre-menstrual tension, Solicitor 6 argued that much would depend on the seriousness of the alleged offence. For a serious offence, such an avenue would need to be explored:

> But you can't use the same argument over a Yorkie bar. On paper, as an academic exercise, I think it is just as right and important that the right decision is made, but at the practical level – and that's what your client is interested in – he's not interested in *mens rea* or *actus reus* – he wants you to get the best result for him [sic] – and sometimes it's not going to be all that easy to get the lady doctor from London to come down and give her menstrual research for a stolen Yorkie bar. In a way it's not right, because if she's not guilty, she's not guilty, but the number of adjournments, the times she'd have to see the doctor and probably have to share with her confidences that she might not be pleased to share....I think, at the end of the day, we've got to weigh it all up and ask, 'Well are we just

causing more trouble?' Put it to her, by all means, but if she says no, then I think you've got to accept that. In a way, maybe she knows what's best for herself.

Most of the solicitors I spoke to, however, saw the presentation of a 'medical' mitigation (as opposed to defence) as one legitimate way of 'playing to the audience'.

I would say that there is more often a 'medical' aspect to the case involving a female offender rather than in the case of a male offender.

(Solicitor 5)

So many of the shoplifting cases involve women and follow the same pattern (middle-aged, on nerve tablets, mind on other things, no previous convictions)...so many of the women who are defendants are at that time of life when it is felt that reports ought to be obtained to establish their needs.

(Solicitor 2)

Thus, despite solicitors' explicit recognition of the material and economic determinants of much female crime, the myth that criminal women are mentally ill, emotionally disturbed, or in some other way abnormal is tenacious. Solicitor 8 gave me this succinct advice:

Be suspicious of women who say they don't need help.

His belief that 'women are more ready to see psychiatrists than men' confirms Gibbens, Soothill, and Pope's finding (1977: 64-5) that psychiatrists regarded women on bail as more amenable than men. By comparison with men remanded on bail, women were rated 'as much less hostile, somewhat less sullen, more anxious and friendly and willing to discuss their problems' (ibid.). This could be accounted for by the fact that the woman offender 'is more likely to seem alarmed and to appeal for help to the psychiatrist, especially if he is a man' (ibid.). The picture is very different, however, if the woman is in custody. She may still seem alarmed but this is now manifested in anger and irritability, 'showing much more violence to staff and other inmates than do male offenders'. Gibbens et al. reflect that this 'clearly highlights the problem of whether one obtains a truer picture of *basic characteristics* during an interview in custody, or on bail' (1977: 65 – emphasis added). Less positivistically, it seems to raise the question of the extent to which custodial remands contribute towards the construction of mental disorder.

Solicitor 8 prided himself on obtaining psychiatric reports from a particular psychiatrist (Doctor A) prior to a court hearing to avoid defendants being remanded in custody, his reasoning being that:

> Only the scum of the medical profession works in prisons – interviews consist of shouting through the door, 'Are you all right?'

This particular solicitor had a very high reputation with defendants and probation officers (confirmed by my interview with Pauline) for 'caring' about female defendants. Even when prosecuting, he often 'slipped in' cases involving women when press reporters were having tea-breaks so that the risk of publicity was minimized, or would openly ask them not to report a case (and usually succeed). He was the epitome of Pollak's 'chivalrous' man yet, ironically, it could be argued that the outcome he obtained for his women clients was not always to their advantage, for he claimed that magistrates always followed Doctor A's recommendations (which usually included some form of treatment). Yet we have seen in the preceding chapter that magistrates are sceptical of psychiatrists and this particular psychiatrist enjoyed a very mixed reputation in the courts. One can only surmise, therefore, that it was the solicitor's eloquence and high standing that achieved results and that consequently his female clients were more likely to end up receiving psychiatric treatment than were the clients of his colleagues.

Other solicitors were less eager to obtain medical reports prior to a request by the court, partly because of the risk of not being able to reclaim the expense through Legal Aid (a risk, as we have seen, which might be greater with women than men) and partly because of a fear of miscalculating the effect of presenting a medical mitigation. The danger of 'taking a sledge-hammer to crack a nut' was voiced by a number of solicitors and this was associated with the embarrassment that a woman was expected to experience at having to declare such problems. One solicitor said he was prepared to use the word 'menopause' but felt unhappy about spelling out any more details:

AW: Is it the mystique of the term that proves a better
defence than spelling out a woman's emotional
and social conditions – how she *feels*?

Solicitor 4: Possibly. You certainly get less questioning by using
the medical terms. Would the client appreciate
being emotionally exposed in the way you suggest?

AW: You mean there's a danger of 'overkill'?

Solicitor 4: Exactly. But I take your point. The best mitigation
for a first offender is to stress the shattering effect
of court proceedings, the humiliation of family
and friends knowing – and that's true – so, in a
way, I suppose you shouldn't need anything else.

A number of issues are conflated in this exchange. First, there
is an acceptance of the power of particular (preferably medical)
words – a power which may be reduced if the word is deconstructed and its components made explicit. This accords with the paradoxical attitude of magistrates to experts which was demonstrated
in the preceding chapter. The use of over-technical language may
be rejected by magistrates as 'unrealistic' and mystifying. On the
other hand, the use of 'common-sense' language can be seen as
insulting, on the grounds that 'we don't need an expert to tell us
that'. Steering a course between the presentation of new,
unfamiliar knowledge which is threatening, and appearing merely
to restate what is 'always and already' known is the solicitor's
particular skill. Second, there is an (unacknowledged) concern
that while medicine has the authority to provide a defence to an
allegation of crime, social and economic conditions have only had
conferred on them the authority sometimes to mitigate punishment. By tailoring his representation to the woman's circumstances and assumed sensitivities, the solicitor overlooks the
possibility that she may, in law, be innocent. He appears to prefer
the compromise of removing the woman from the more
contentious site of medical explanation and relocating her in the
site of familial need, while retaining her status as hapless, guilt-
ridden victim of her own uncontrollable impulses. Additionally,
family and friends are portrayed as the 'real' sufferers, who have
been betrayed by this woman, rather than as the possible source
of her misery – the constraints and pressures against which she
may be protesting.

The pressure on a woman to construct an explanation of her action which will appease her family was recognized by Solicitor 6, who argued that solicitors had to assess the consequences of colluding with such a course. The myth of 'providing a service' and 'taking instructions' remains, and solicitors were reluctant to acknowledge the extent to which they control the staging of women's representation:

> You've always got to remember just how far your lady is
> prepared to go. She may feel that it is far more degrading to go
> into a witness box and tell them all those type of details than to
> just get it over. Quite regularly all they want to do is get it over
> anyway – they don't think about the weight of the conviction –
> and I think you've got to respect their wishes and if they are
> not prepared to bare their private lives for what they class as a
> very minor matter, and one which they feel they can somehow
> square with the family, then they could always go away and say,
> 'I didn't really want to talk about all those details' which gives
> them a safety net as well. You see quite often it's not 'Well I
> admitted that I was responsible for this' but 'I admitted it but it
> was just to save myself telling them all those other bits'. So in
> those circumstances, they wouldn't find it such a pressing need
> to weigh up the differences. If it's a more serious matter, like
> murder, you have to put a bit more pressure on them and say,
> 'When you look at what you're facing, your embarrassment
> about your menstrual cycle pales into insignificance – you've
> got to pull yourself together and fight for this.'

This would again seem to confirm Edwards's suggestion (1984: 197) 'that the nature of the offence for which a defendant is charged is likely to have a considerable impact on whether or not a medical report is requested'.

Elsewhere (Worrall 1981), I have argued that 'medical' mitigations in respect of female law-breakers rarely claim to be concerned with clinically definable mental illness. Apart from references to 'depression' most solicitors seemed to associate medical reports and psychiatric treatment with gynaecological conditions which are arguably 'normal' – pre-menstrual tension, pregnancy, the menopause. In other words, the normal woman is likely to be viewed as abnormal. But the extent to which such abnormality should be considered to excuse criminal behaviour is a legal dilemma which is exemplified in the development of the 'reasonable man' test (Allen 1987b). In the case of Camplin (1978), Lord Simon Glaisdale argued that, while the term 'reasonable man' must be assumed to include 'the reasonable woman', the jury must be precluded 'from considering that the accused was, say, pregnant' or, presumably, undergoing menstruation or menopause. Such conditions, it was maintained, must fall into the category of 'personal idiosyncrasy' rather than 'universal quality'. In 1982 when the case of Smith alias Craddock eventually reached the Court of Appeal, it was decided that pre-menstrual tension 'was "wholly unacceptable" as a defence to any crime. Under British law evidence of PMT can only be introduced as an extenuating factor or in mitigation of sentence....(1982 CLR 531)' (Edwards 1984: 85).

The degree, therefore, to which the 'reasonable man' recognizes the 'normal woman' is dependent not on the strength of proof of any antecedent condition but on the material consequences of that recognition. If 'feminine conditions' are recognized only in mitigation and not in defence, then their recognition assists the *management* of female law-breakers without conceding authority (or, indeed, authenticity) to the women's own accounts.

CONCLUSION

Solicitors constitute an important link in the chain of the socio-legal signification of women law-breakers. By re-presenting the woman to the court, they are concerned both to protect the woman from her own tendencies to present herself in an 'unacceptable' way and to 'normalize' the woman and her actions so that she and they may be presented in a form that is 'recognized' by the court. In carrying out this task, solicitors are mindful of certain rules and conventions governing their representation. The woman's story must be packaged in such a way that her plea of 'guilty' is received without discomfort by the court and her own account of events must be reconstituted or muted. She herself is disqualified as a speaker of her own story and a certain 'hierarchy of credibility' pertains to the explanations offered for offences that can be categorized as 'serious but natural' (i.e., congruent with images of femininity) or 'petty but unnatural', and committed by 'respectable' women. 'Need' is an acceptable explanation if the offence is 'petty but natural' and if such an explanation does not imply that 'society' (as represented by the court) is to blame. Poverty *per se* is never an acceptable explanation. Offences which are either 'serious and unnatural' or 'petty and unnatural' are likely to be explained in terms of 'greed' or wickedness, especially if committed by 'unrespectable' women, namely, working-class women or women with so-called unconventional lifestyles.

In order to secure the best possible position in that hierarchy for their clients, but without damaging their own professional credibility, solicitors adopt a strategy which is ostensibly characterized by the paradigm of 'service'. By using the vocabulary of service ('client', 'taking instructions', etc.) solicitors perpetuate the myth of defendant choice and power. Because of the material and ideological constraints on women in society, such vocabulary is particularly ironic in relation to female law-breakers.

Within this context, solicitors employ a variety of tactics which include: recognizing when gender-related explanations may or may not be acceptable; the stance of moral neutrality (which renders the 'truth' of an account irrelevant and avoids the need to recognize gender-related injustices); 'getting to know the Bench'; and 'playing to the audience' – all of which tactics involve simultaneously acknowledging and reinforcing ideologies about the 'normal' woman.

Underpinning these ideological conditions governing the relationship between solicitors and female defendants is the economic condition of women's particularly precarious ability to pay for legal representation. The readiness of solicitors to utilize 'off the peg', ready-made packages for women law-breakers may be attributed as much to economic as to ideological considerations.

Thus, solicitors construct female law-breakers within the ideologies of domesticity, sexuality, and pathology. Women defendants are re-presented as family members, as sexual objects, and/or as sick. Even those for whom such constructions bear no relation to reality cannot escape the power of these ideologies. Their only alternative is to be constructed in terms of their exclusion from these 'socially exculpatory' and 'legally effective' (Edwards 1984) categories. It has been argued that these categories emanate from a socio-legal belief in the fundamental 'normality' of *man*. They constitute concessions to those defendants who suffer the misfortune of being *non-male*. Exclusion from these categories, therefore, renders the 'nondescript' female law-breaker neither *male* nor *non-male*. Thus we return to Lombroso's monstrous 'double exception' (Lambroso and Ferrero 1959).

Chapter Six

TREATABLE WOMEN?

Identifying the gender-specific implications of the rules governing psychiatrists' discourse is a task which is both easy and elusive. It is easy in the sense that, since women dominate the official statistics of psychiatric treatment, it could be argued that the rules outlined earlier in this study are applied routinely primarily to women rather than men. As Allen (1986: 85) observes, 'the female is not the "special" but the normal form of the psychiatric patient'. On the other hand, medicine, like law, views itself as 'gender-neutral'. With the marginalized exception of dysfunctions emanating from gynaecological disorders, its categories do not recognize distinctions of gender *per se.* Exposing the 'unspoken "she" of psychiatry...behind the bland "he" of the psychiatric textbooks' (Allen 1986: 87) is, therefore, a difficult task, especially if one wishes to avoid the pitfall of arguing that there exists a 'patriarchal complicity in the apparent mental morbidity of women', which is constitutive of psychiatry (rather than contingent to it) – an argument which Allen (1986) persuasively demonstrates to be untenable.

Despite this dilemma, it is possible to identify from the information obtained from the psychiatrists in this study some indications of specific mechanisms which permit them to describe most of their female patients as 'normal' women (that is, with a 'normal' propensity for sickness). Those mechanisms, however, serve concomitantly to ensure that the particular women in this study are excluded from that category and are thus rendered nondescript.

THE CONSTRUCTION OF ORDERED WOMEN

Recognizable paradigms

Some psychiatrists acknowledged that they and their colleagues might be committed to different 'models' of mental illness and that this would materially affect their diagnoses and interventions:

> There are two basic schools of psychiatry – those who believe that a psychotic illness is medical and those who believe that it is an extension of something else. I happen to be towards the behaviour model rather than the medical model, and I talk about schizophrenogenic situations rather than somebody who has got something wrong with their midbrain. So you have to start by knowing what sort of a person I am professionally.
>
> (Dr C)

Certain paradigms were also seen to be more acceptable to courts than others:

> If you use terms like 'depression', 'obsession', and 'schizophrenia' you don't get cross-examined, but if you start using psychoanalytical terms, talking about a 'subconscious wish to be punished', that's not acceptable. I had a woman recently who was fined for shoplifting, but went out and did it again immediately – as though she wanted more punishment. But you can't say that in a report.
>
> (Dr D)

The prohibition of psychoanalytical discourse from the utterances of psychiatrists in court could be viewed as having a gender-specific effect on the assessment of female law-breakers. Psychoanalysis *can* be viewed as a challenge to the clinical model of psychiatry and, as such, has been used by feminists to offer 'alternative' therapy to women (Eichenbaum and Orbach 1982). Despite the limitations of feminist therapy (Allen 1986), its exclusion from 'respectable' psychiatric diagnosis places yet one more restriction on the range of categories within which female law-breakers can legitimately be described.

One psychiatrist who admitted to working psychoanalytically (Dr C) suggested that there was an additional dimension of class

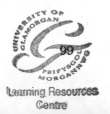

to this restriction. He believed that the female law-breakers that he saw were likely to be from social classes 3, 4, and 5, whereas:

> We have a professional department (nearby) where they head their letters 'Forensic Psychiatry' and all that sort of thing. Your polite (middle-class) lady who is filling her knickers with goodies from Woolies is likely to be sent to very proper psychiatrists elsewhere, whereas hack psychiatrists like myself wouldn't see her.

It would appear possible to infer from this that the effectiveness of paradigms differs according to the social class of the referred woman. The 'respectable', 'middle-class' woman may be described as 'depressed' (clinical model) and treatable by drug therapy – that is, capable of being 'rendered undepressed' (Dr A). Alternatively, she may be described in terms of her 'cry for help', 'sense of guilt', and her 'wish to be punished' or to 'commit social suicide' (psychoanalytical model). Such a description will normally be made within a relationship of benevolent paternalism:

> Many would prefer to be in prison. We're too kind here – no structure. But it would be irrational to punish in those circumstances, wouldn't it?
>
> (Dr E)

For such women, the vocabulary of punishment can be introduced as safely symbolic. For the working-class woman, however, there is a real danger that courts may take it literally and that the answer to Dr E's rhetorical question may turn out to be a resounding 'No'.

The invocation of conflicting paradigms of mental illness also poses difficulties when deciding the appropriateness of referrals to psychiatrists. Nurse A (a community psychiatric nurse) was not convinced that the right people were being referred:

> What tends to happen is that we get people referred for what I would say are the wrong reasons and the wrong type of people, i.e., the type of problems that I would say I could deal with best tend not to get referred. This is often a fault of people not being assessed properly in the first place. Things like neurosis – a lot of people wouldn't identify it as neurosis. A patient might go along to a GP complaining of aches and pains or irritable –

complaining of the signs and symptoms of anxiety or stress –
and there's a tendency that it's treated with tablets, rather than
sitting down and looking at why is the person like this – it's not
an illness – why is the person *behaving* like this. People tend not
to get referred for this kind of reason – they are referred
because they are *ill*, whatever that means....

(Nurse A)

Because the parameters of what might constitute mental illness
(and hence an 'appropriate' referral) are drawn so widely, it
becomes essential within psychiatric discourse that there exist a
person with unchallenged authority to decide what does constitute
mental illness in any given case. The turning of a collection of
disparate symptoms into the intelligible signs of a disease by the
trained gaze of a doctor is central to the task of clinical analysis. As
Foucault (1973) argues, the indispensable power of the doctor to
describe a disease emerged in the eighteenth century when medical
science began to reject the 'essential' paradigm of disease (that is,
the belief that there existed an 'ideal form' of disease, whose whole
was greater than the sum of its symptomatic parts). In its place was
established a paradigm within which 'symptoms do not by
themselves announce the disease: they are turned into intelligible
signs...by a trained observer' (Cousins and Hussain 1984: 160).

The gender-specific implication of this is that many of the
qualities ascribed to the 'normal' woman are also viewed as
constituting 'intelligible signs' of mental disorder. When to this is
added the statistical abnormality of female law-breaking, the
relationship between criminal activity and mental disorder in
women seems over-determined. Dr B explained that approximately 25 per cent of the referrals his forensic unit received were
women. In reply to my comment that this seemed high in comparison with their rate of offending, he said:

Yes, but as you are aware, they have a higher psychiatric
morbidity – or are thought to have. In fact, relatively few get
into trouble....When they do, it's because they are a very
disturbed group.

In the light of such comments, it is unsurprising that most of
the psychiatrists viewed most of the referrals of female law-
breakers as 'appropriate':

101

When a woman offends, the usual reaction is 'I wonder what's wrong with her'. When a man offends, it's a different reaction. So in that respect the referrals are appropriate, in so far as everyone is worrying about what has gone wrong with this poor woman!

(Dr C)

Women usually do suffer from treatable disorders – usually depression. They suffer more functional disorders than men – with men it's more inadequacy, low intelligence, and drink.

(Dr D)

Yet, having said that most referrals of women were appropriate, psychiatrists still reserved the right subsequently to redefine those same symptoms as being beyond their competence to treat:

The women I see at (the probation hostel)... almost without exception are, loosely, personality disorders or rather late developing adolescents, rather than being psychotic or severely mentally ill. But occasionally the staff there find their behaviour so bizarre or worrying that *they* wonder whether they are psychotic. But I don't think I've found a psychotic person there for two years now.

(Dr C)

Diagnosis is very important for women. There are far fewer of them offending – that's a cultural thing – but they are much worse. Very few offenders are mentally ill – many have personality disorders.

(Dr F)

I would have said...about 50 per cent of the women either don't suffer from a treatable mental disorder or the disorder is in the form of psychopathic traits, or personality disorder, and in that event it's a moot point whether there is treatment as such.

(Dr A)

Redefining sickness as neediness

In psychiatric discourse the notion of 'treatability' has been turned on its head. In order to render themselves treatable, potential patients have to satisfy certain social criteria. Conversely, if psychiatrists decide that they will not or cannot treat a defendant, they can redefine the symptoms of mental disorder as symptoms of something else – in particular, as symptoms of social, rather than medical need.   The consequence has been that psychiatrists have partially appropriated the paradigm of 'anti-psychiatry' while failing to vacate the site of privilege which is an essential precondition of that discourse They have claimed the right to redefine mental illness as 'problems of living' (Szasz 1973) but have not simultaneously disqualified themselves as expert speakers. On the contrary, they have transferred their expertise to a competing discourse – that of social work. Only one psychiatrist appeared to appreciate the irony of adopting this position:

> 'Is it to this man's disadvantage to go to prison?' I don't like being asked that. It's to everyone's disadvantage but it isn't any more important coming from a psychiatrist. I used to think I could do everyone's job – I'm learning my limitations as I get older.

> (Dr D)

But even Dr D still considered himself competent to enter social work discourse by making recommendations that defendants would 'benefit from the support of a sympathetic probation officer'.

Psychiatrists retain their power as overseers of social work in the criminal justice system by redefining evidence of sickness as evidence of neediness. The specific mechanism employed in relation to the nondescript woman is that, having been defined as an 'appropriate' referral for psychiatric assessment, she is then constructed *by psychiatric discourse* not within the discourse of pathology but within the discourses of domesticity and sexuality. She is described as needing not psychiatric but social work intervention. Dr F's assessment of Maureen (taken from her file) illustrates the point:

> I am more convinced every day that her problem is basically a marital one. I think that, as a psychiatrist, I have very little to offer this lady. Most of her problems are social ones.

As has been seen, one of the ways in which psychiatrists redefine female law-breakers is by arguing that they are personality disordered rather than being 'really' mentally ill. A second way, however, is to redefine dysfunctions arising from gynaecological disorders as being 'just' forms of stress. If magistrates and solicitors are sceptical of explanations that attribute criminal behaviour to such disorders so, too, it seems, are psychiatrists:

> I think that this is a fashionable bandwagon to jump on to and that PMT – where it exists – is simply another form of stress. You can be depressed with PMT and shoplift or break your child's arm or you can get depressed and break your child's arm because you have arthritis or because your husband's out drinking. I don't think, by and large, it differs from any other form of serious stress and, of course, when you write a report and there are extenuating circumstances – things you think should be considered in sentencing, not when considering guilt – then it is fair to say, 'This woman is depressed because of PMT, or she has arthritis or her husband is always beating her or whatever....' It's just a form of stress.
>
> (Dr A)

> I have a few cases where shoplifting has been associated with pre-menstrual tension - not very many. I think it is occasionally and rather rarely associated with uncharacteristic behaviour. It's not common. It's been vastly overrated in the last year or two in its importance. I've had a few rare cases - a murder case - I seem to remember that the woman was controlled on hormonal drugs and she wasn't taking them. It was known that in the pre-menstrual phase she used to behave very strangely and aggressively and that was a case of significance. But I wouldn't put the explanation in terms of PMT, but rather in terms of mental and emotional disturbance that happens at that time, one of the causes of which might be pre-menstrual tension. But I think it's asking for trouble to try to explain it away simply on PMT. It's just rare cases where it has very bizarre effects - but in relation to the number of people who suffer from PMT it's insignificant.
>
> (Dr B)

Dr B is recognized as an authority on infanticide and his

expressed views therefore both reflect and reinforce judicial attitudes:

> The wording of the Infanticide Act (1938) requires it to be shown that the woman suffered from a disturbance of the mind due to the fact that she had not fully recovered from the effects of childbirth or lactation and I think there is perhaps a slight hardening of view that it was not because they had not recovered from childbirth or lactation but that they suffered from depression anyway - then it would be dealt with as manslaughter, although the outcome will be the same It's rare for them to be sent to prison - they're nearly always put on probation.

The substitution of socio-economic discourse (in particular, the vocabulary of 'stress') for gynaecological discourse might be welcomed by some feminists. For instance, Susan Edwards (1984) has argued that female law-breakers should resist attempts to reduce their behaviour to their biology. Yet, as O'Donovan (1984) has indicated, such changes of orientation among professionals still raise problems for women. The removal of gender-related *Biology* excusing conditions in the face of continuing material inequality *should* between the sexes may increase rather than reduce discriminatory *not be* practices. The argument that 'men, too, are subject to the social *ignored* stresses of rearing children, particularly if unsupported by women' (Edwards 1984: 96) does not logically invalidate the differential treatment of women in circumstances that are materially and specifically different (after all, men do not produce babies and if a woman says childbirth has certain effects on her, why should that statement be declared self-evidently invalid?). Equally, while child-rearing is undoubtedly stressful for both men and women, in reality the 'unsupported' father is likely to receive more sympathy in any case than the 'unsupported' mother, who is presumed to have 'natural resources' of 'maternal instincts' to help her survive adverse social conditions (Dominelli 1984: 101). The substitution of one discourse for another does not necessarily alter the power relationship between the describer and the described, nor does it guarantee any greater degree of control by women over their own destiny. Psychiatrists still arrogate to themselves competence to explain female law-breaking behaviour and to judge culpability as well as treatability.

Ironically, women who are accepted as being 'treatable' are often viewed as using domestic 'stress' as an excuse for not co-operating. As has been seen, psychiatrists tend to view female law-breakers as 'unreliable' about keeping appointments. At the Special Treatment Unit,[1] one of the nurses told me:

> Most women are here for marital problems, alcohol or drug abuse (that is, usually prescribed drugs). They are no particular problem on the Unit, although some use their children as an excuse for not settling.

Nurse B felt that:

> Women could use the Unit more but they don't really want to make the decisions that will change their situations.

Dr F echoed this:

> Women use domestic responsibilities as an excuse for not coming into the Unit – they look for any excuse to avoid *the issue.*

(my emphasis)

Women, therefore, are blamed for not seeing 'the issue' as being that which psychiatrists describe as being 'the issue'. But this is hardly surprising, since the women so described have in reality been set yet another trap. Their attempts to demonstrate their maternal competence to the court are now used in evidence against them - apparently indicating a lack of co-operation, an unwillingness to undertake 'treatment'. The dilemma is further compounded when one begins to consider the 'treatment'.

TREATING WOMEN

The Unit is run on the lines of a therapeutic community, which means regular group meetings and patients are allowed to go home at weekends. The average stay, according to Dr F

> if they survive the first week, is about two months – sometimes four.

Such an experience would appear to be well-suited to the needs of women who might otherwise be at risk of imprisonment, provided they could make the necessary child-care arrangements. However, there was evidence that the regime in the Unit served to reproduce the very familial roles which patients had, for one reason or another, found intolerable outside:

> You couldn't get a greater mix of social misfits, but it works. There's no great secret – it's just like an extended family – we play family roles...

> (Nurse B)

What happens at the Special Treatment Unit is therefore located both discursively and physically (weekdays spent in hospitals, weekends at home) at the interstices of medico-psychiatric, familial, and penal discourse. The expectation that, as 'social misfits', they can nevertheless be 'fitted' into family roles in a medical setting to which they have been sent by a judicial authority reproduces for female law-breakers the very descriptive trap which they have sought, through their law-breaking, to avoid. It seems, therefore, that whatever benefit women might obtain from the experience of communal living provided at the Unit will continue to be limited by its discursive location and the very real material problems of retaining a 'weekend home' and being a 'weekend mother'.

It could be argued that at the Special Treatment Unit psychiatry has laid claim to what is basically an experiment in communal living. Nevertheless, here, as with all psychiatric treatment ordered by a criminal court, it seems to be professionals other than psychiatrists who carry the main responsibility. Psychiatry's desire to oversee social work has two consequences for probation officers.

First, probation officers frequently have to accept recommendations for probation made by psychiatrists. The following are by no means uncommon recommendations in psychiatrists' reports:

> In my opinion, and with respect to the court, should she be found guilty of the offence with which she is charged, her best interests might be served by close and strict probationary supervision.

> (Unknown psychiatrist reporting on Jean, who, at this stage, had not even been found guilty)

I feel the family as a whole could be helped a great deal by an experienced probation officer or social worker.

(Dr A reporting on a client of Probation Officer 15)

From my interviews with probation officers, it was evident that Dr A had, over the years, enraged generations of probation officers by persistently claiming expertise in assessing suitability for probation.

Dr B assured me that his relationship with probation officers was very much 'a team matter':

I would never make a recommendation for probation without talking to the probation officer – I would never make a recommendation against the probation officer's view – it's quite inappropriate.

Nevertheless, one probation officer recounted with delight an incident in which Dr B had done precisely that and had been challenged by a magistrate:

He had suggested probation with a condition of psychiatric treatment. The stipendiary magistrate – bless his cotton socks! – had said, 'That's all very well, Dr B, but shall we let probation have a look at it?'

(Probation Officer 5)

Psychiatry has the power to intrude into a discourse which is not its own (namely, the discourse of social work) and to appropriate in the name of 'consultancy' both the paradigms of social, rather than medical, neediness and the personnel of social work. The following remarks by Dr A illustrate the extent to which probation officers are viewed by psychiatrists as providing a service for the benefit of psychiatry:

Basically, I would have said that going into the Probation Service is not something that is very prestigious, on the one hand, or likely to make your fortune, on the other. And therefore I would have thought that nine out of ten probation officers are into this because they want to help and are enthusiastic. In the main, they are very co-operative – I find them very helpful people to deal with. Just occasionally, I find that the information they come up with is a little thin but then some of them have enormous caseloads and not much time to do it...By and large, I am struck by the frequency with which they come to the same conclusion as mine, quite independently.

Magistrates and probation officers often interpret this congruity of conclusion as being more indicative of a lack of expertise on the part of psychiatrists than of any unexpected medical expertise on the part of probation officers. Nevertheless, psychiatrists arrogate to themselves the right to assess defendants and view probation officers' 'knowledge' in this area as being inferior in the sense that it exists to reinforce psychiatric discourse. When it comes to treatment, however, probation officers find that their expertise is elevated and afforded greater respect.

The second consequence of psychiatric oversight is that psychiatrists appear to defer to probation officers' greater expertise in the management of the mentally disordered.

There is evidence (Gibbens, Soothill, and Pope 1977) that, once psychiatrists have made their assessments, they are not conspicuously enthusiastic about carrying out their recommendations, especially if, as in recommendations for probation orders with conditions of treatment, these are supposed to involve joint work with probation officers. Psychiatrists show a reluctance to become over-involved in 'court order' cases because, as Lewis (1980: 26) observes, 'the notion of "enforced compliance" upsets some psychiatrists':

> I am often reluctant to treat people who are subject to court orders as I feel that for the patient to benefit he has to be committed to his treatment...I have not noticed any difference between men and women with regard to this.
>
> (Dr G)

> Most patients on court orders I see only once in two or three months – and I stand by for emergencies. I think the probation officer does most of the work – I just support and monitor progress.
>
> (Dr E)

In Kathy's case, Dr A apparently felt under no obligation to see a woman convicted of manslaughter at all, even though he had given an undertaking to a Crown Court that he would see her. Kathy killed her sister and was convicted of manslaughter on the grounds of diminished responsibility, having been remanded in custody and given an EEG test, the results of which were abnormal. The prison doctor had felt that this required further investigation and treatment and, at court, Dr A had agreed to see Kathy as an out-patient. Directly as a result of this undertaking, the judge embarked on the 'exceptional course' of placing her on probation. She was never seen by Dr A. Once Kathy had been rendered harmless by psychiatric assessment (Allen 1987a), treatment was presumably unnecessary and she could be left safely in the hands of the Probation Service.

Probation officers felt that psychiatrists were often indifferent and egocentric. Co-operation, on the occasions when it was identified, was treasured as a rare commodity, usually won through hard-fought battles or teeth-gritting sycophancy. Two cases illustrated these points vividly.

Mandy, a woman who had asked magistrates to send her to prison (see Chapter 7), was later convicted of arson with intent to endanger life, an offence which can carry a life sentence. At the Crown Court, Dr F reported that she was 'a psychopathic personality...too dangerous for him to admit to his clinic and he had made arrangements for the forensic psychiatrist from Broadmoor to interview her' (recounted by Probation Officer 20). The probation officer felt that this recommendation was too extreme and that there must be other places Mandy could go to. The solicitor agreed and promptly sought a second opinion from another psychiatrist:

> He wrote a report saying that she was a psychopathic
> personality, that prison would do no good for her, certainly
> Special Hospital would do no good for her and as he didn't
> know of any other hospitals that would be interested,
> probation in the community was the best thing he could
> suggest. So we'd got two psychiatrists, the second doing a
> whitewash at the request of the solicitors who were paying him
> privately – not that I can ever prove that!

As has been seen, psychiatrists routinely invoke the rules of

110

'treatability' to legitimate the non-treatment of defendants diagnosed as suffering from psychopathic disorders. The barrister subsequently tried to persuade the probation officer to endorse the recommendation for probation and, when the latter refused the request, refused to submit any psychiatric reports at all. The probation officer continued:

> I felt she needed hospital treatment but it seemed that the community was not prepared to provide any of the resources that this sort of person requires. I left it at that and she got a three-year sentence.

Gwen's offence of throwing a brick through her own window hardly put her in the same league as Mandy. The magistrates, however, wanted a psychiatric report and were threatening to remand her in custody in order to obtain it. Probation Officer 2, who was on court duty that day, was concerned about this, discovered that Gwen had received psychiatric treatment in the past, and set about contacting the local psychiatric hospital. When she eventually got through to the appropriate consultant, the following conversation ensued:

> So I say, 'Gwen X – is she known to you?' 'Ah yes', he said, 'What's the trouble?' I said, 'She committed this offence – it's only a minor offence, but the magistrates want medical reports and it means that unless you can take her, she will go to prison.' So there's silence at the end of the phone. 'And why do you think she shouldn't go to prison, Mrs C? Don't you think it might do her good?' I was so horrified at this that I said, 'No I don't think it will do her good.' I forgot for a minute that I was speaking to this God-like man. 'I see one of my tasks as keeping the inappropriate out of prison and I actually think this lady is inappropriate.' And he started to laugh and he said, 'I just wanted to see whether you had a good reason.'

The stories of Gwen and Mandy illustrate the iatrogenic nature of their treatment. Both were subject to properly authorized welfare intervention yet their nondescriptiveness had over-determined their failure. The discourses within which they had been constructed had failed to legitimate the Other of their own definitions of reality and had thus provided for them a definitional trap into which they could not fit but from which they could not escape. Victims of the system's inability to categorize them, they had, in reality, been set up to fail. In this situation, probation officers frequently saw themselves as hostages to fortune, the provision of the 1983 Mental Health Act that hospital admission should only take place when treatment is available having been turned on its head to sanction psychiatrists making their actual diagnoses of mental illness fit the available treatment.

'There is nothing we can do for her; therefore, there is nothing wrong.' I'm afraid I've got a bad impression of [psychiatrists]. If they don't think they can do anything, they say there is nothing wrong [and] they recommend a probation order.

(Probation Officer 11)

The dilemma facing probation officers was clearly expounded by Probation Officer 3 in a discussion about the Special Treatment Unit. On the one hand, he was sceptical both about the treatment on offer, which was based on 'keeping people talking', and about the very brief time that people were required to be resident:

In the nicest possible way, they are just waffle groups. Now that can be very useful over perhaps a year, but in a couple of weeks, what good does it do anybody?

On the other hand, he felt compelled to make use of the facility for two reasons:

One is the possibility that she could get treatment that I couldn't possibly give her – the feeling that I can't handle this, it is *way* beyond me...There is a cry for help – from me – about what to do with the case. The other is a ploy, because you know that even if the treatment does her no good at all, providing she spends a respectable amount of time there, it's not too painful for her and it's a lot less bad than prison.

In other words, he felt the need to work strategically. But ploys have a nasty habit of backfiring, especially if there are any further court appearances:

I think what they'll view her as is someone who's been given the best help available in the area and failed to use it...The recommendation is two-edged in that it saves them this time but will crucify them next time.

112

CONCLUSION

Forensic psychiatrists make a unique contribution to the 'chain of signification' of female law-breakers by constructing them as treatable (or not), not only within psychiatric discourse but also within social work and penal discourse. The origin of psychiatrists' transferable authority rests on their paradoxical relationship with other court-room personnel. The legally defined powers of psychiatrists to assess, judge, and manage law-breakers are wide-ranging but entirely discretionary. The invocation of these powers is dependent on the extent to which psychiatrists and other personnel are prepared to enter into a descriptive and prescriptive collusion in relation to the organization of the difference which constitutes the 'culpable/not culpable' and 'treatment/ punishment' distinctions.

It has been argued that the women in this study have been muted by psychiatrists because they have been subject to a formal psychiatry which purports to be essentially gender-neutral but which they have experienced as being substantively discriminatory. The gap between the ideological claims of psychiatric discourse and the range of unlegitimated interpretations of women's behaviour which they seek to contain is foreclosed in a number of ways.

1) By invoking the female domination of the official statistics of mental illness to demonstrate that even 'normal' women are prone to mental instability, those women who deviate from normal gender expectations by breaking the law are viewed as doubly prone to such instability.

2) By invoking a clinical paradigm of mental illness, most psychiatrists are committed to the use of restricted and rigid categories of diagnosis which are frequently experienced as incongruent with the lived realities of these women. Alternative paradigms which construct mental illness as the product of unresolved internal conflict (psychoanalysis) and/or problems of living (anti-psychiatry) are largely ejected from the site of assessment because they represent the Other which threatens authorized wisdom.

3) By invoking and then turning on its head the notion of 'treatability', psychiatrists claim authority to redefine evidence of sickness in these women as evidence of neediness. This is

113

demonstrated in two particular ways. First, those who deviate from 'normal' femininity are constructed as having personality disorders rather than being 'really' mentally ill. Second, those who suffer gynaecologically based disorders are redefined as being 'just' subject to a particular form of stress (which is itself deemed to be gender-neutral).

Consequently, nondescript women fall both within and without the domain of psychiatry. Psychiatrists retain their authority to assess and judge them but, by redefining their 'sickness' as neediness, they simultaneously deny responsibility for treating them. Despite this, they retain their oversight of those social workers and probation officers whom they then charge with the women's 'treatment'.

Chapter Seven

MANAGEABLE WOMEN?

The 'Alternatives to Custody' debate has been constructed within probation discourse in such a way as to ensure that it both ignores and is irrelevant to female law-breakers. This is not because women are not sent to prison; clearly they are – and in increasing numbers (Home Office 1986a). But the current debate ignores the complexity of the route that leads them there. It does this in two ways. First, it renders the majority of female law-breakers invisible by constructing them as 'not recidivists'. Second, it renders a minority of female law-breakers highly visible by assuming that their presence in prison demonstrates either their dangerousness or their incorrigibility, rather than demonstrating the inadequacy of the discourses within which they are so constructed. This study demonstrates that increasing numbers of female law-breakers are trapped by a judicial need to fit them into one or other of these categories.

As has been seen, the 'programme' through which probation officers assess or categorize defendants in ways which are recognizable to courts is the social inquiry report. Although this study has not specifically examined reports on women, it has sought to offer an analysis of the discourses within which they – and psychiatric reports – are authorized, written, and received (that is, read and acted upon or rejected). It has been argued that female law-breakers are rendered 'programmable' (that is, presented as in need of, motivated towards, and capable of benefiting from the resources of the Probation Service) through their construction within the discourses of domesticity, sexuality, and pathology. The trap for probation officers who might want to construct female law-breakers within alternative discourses is that, in an area where such stereotypes dominate, they run the risk of seriously disadvantaging their client. Hence many officers justify their continued writing of gender-stereotyped reports on the grounds that they are working tactically in their clients' best interests.

But tactical working does not end in the court-room. This chapter examines the consequences of this 'dissonance trap' for probation officers in their daily work with the nondescript women who are so frequently placed under their supervision. It is argued that, in relation to such women, probation discourse is characterized by:

1) recognition of the contradictory effects of the 'gender contract' – the ideological and material conditions within which many wome 1 clients are located;

2) a sense of frustration/powerlessness, provoked by:

a) the apparently self-destructive contract avoidance behaviour of some women clients and

b) the apparent indifference of professionals, officials, and politicians who are perceived to have the power (that is, the authority plus the expertise/knowledge plus the material resources) to bring about effective change in the lives of these women;

3) an occasional sense of achievement when:

a) in the absence of an alternative discourse within which to work, the contradictions of the gender contract are exploited (through 'working tactically') to the benefit of some women clients (though, inevitably, to the detriment of others?) or

b) some women are enabled to find non-self-destructive 'ways round' the gender contract.

IDENTIFYING THE CONTRADICTORY EFFECTS OF THE GENDER CONTRACT

The starting point of this analysis is a comment made by a male probation officer working in a women's prison. He was asked whether he agreed with the view of a previously interviewed female probation officer that women evade reality more than men and that prison helps them to face up to the consequence of their behaviour. He replied:

For some women, reality is provision for their families. I have found that women in prison are on the whole more realistic than men...and perhaps they suffer more from the fact that *they are rooted in relationships.*

(Probation Officer 8)

Who does and does not have the authority to define what constitutes 'reality' for female law-breakers is one of the central questions which has to be addressed by any analysis of the gender contract. Magistrates, solicitors, psychiatrists, and probation officers claim to have such authority but the women themselves are muted and their definitions of reality subjugated. Being 'rooted' might be translated in authorized discourses as being securely surrounded by conditions conducive to growth but in the women's discourse as being immovably transfixed in a position of some danger (as in 'rooted to the spot').

Most probation officers recognized that many of the women had committed crimes because they were 'desperate' for money and that they could be viewed as 'not really criminal when it comes to the point – not to that extent' (Probation Officer 4 on Eileen). But the relationship between poverty and criminal activity was often more complex than that and this gave rise to attitudes of wariness on the part of would-be sympathizers. Probation Officer 9 explained what happened to Jean on her release from her prison sentence for baby-snatching:

She'd been given a house...by the Housing Department – that had been arranged by the Social Services – and she shoplifted. She shoplifted a baby bath, would you believe, and maternity clothes and a number of other things. The policewoman was very, very sympathetic, until she got back to the house and realized how much other stuff she'd got, which was probably also shoplifted, and I can tell you, I wasn't very nice to her (i.e., to Jean).

Deprived of her own family and punished for snatching someone else's Jean had resorted to 'providing' for her next baby, which she knew was likely to be removed from her at birth. Initially the object of official sympathy, she rapidly became the object of official anger when the extent of her 'provision' became apparent. Yet the conflicting pressures resulting from giving this woman a

117

home and setting up expectations of her as a mother while also planning to deprive her (possibly for very understandable reasons) of that anticipated family do not seem to have been appreciated.

The extent to which the families in which some of the women lived could be held to be actively responsible for some women's criminal activity was also recognized. Lack of appreciation, a sense of injustice, and having to cope with 'chaos' were all proposed as factors precipitating the commission of crimes, particularly by middle-aged and older women. Probation Officer 10 spoke of a widow who chose to plead guilty to shoplifting 'to get it over with', although the officer felt she might have had a defence to the charge:

> It's the saddest case I've ever come across. Her family meant everything to her but they didn't have the same regard for her.

The subsequent probation order provided an opportunity for the probation officer to undertake 'grief counselling' with the woman – a valuable service but, it might be argued, one which should not have required the catalyst of a criminal conviction to obtain. Probation Officer 7 described a woman whose husband had left her for a younger woman. Ethel was on probation for the theft of a chicken valued at £2:

> She's a sad little lady who has just had all the spirit knocked out of her...But she's a very upright woman – she thinks it's terrible that her husband should be allowed...She got herself into a state...and had to sit there and not be able to defend herself about what he'd done to her. And she put her coat on and went out and thought 'Why should I pay for this chicken?'

This apparently irrational behaviour arising from a sense of powerlessness in the face of injustice has been described elsewhere (Carlen 1988: 126) as the 'Sod It' Syndrome, and it is evidently not confined to young, overtly troublesome women. Probation Officer 7 cited a further example of a woman whose crime could be viewed as a response to years of being 'a dish-rack and a door-mat':

> She's now got a grown-up family...and she's going through the unhappiness of the children not supporting her. They don't do

the jobs in the house, they don't help as much as she feels they should. She feels she's providing a home, and why should she?

But perhaps the most vivid description of the damaging effects of the family came from Probation Officer 1 in her discussion of Maureen's chaotic family situation. The following are excerpts from her interview:

> Maureen, although she's cast as the non-coper, is the coper, and she copes by committing offences, to try, in her way, to get them out of trouble. But all she manages to do is get herself into trouble. The family do survive while she's away, and they have very little regard for her really. Maureen's been diagnosed over the years as schizophrenic, personality disordered – it's usually been those sorts of labels that have been bandied about – or 'subject to anxiety attacks'. I mean, I don't know what you do with a label when you've got it. She certainly does get very anxious about things...and she can see that she is over-reacting, but still isn't able to stop over-reacting...The family have gotten almost to 'Oh, she's off again' and collude with each other in isolating Maureen as *the* problem. In effect, the problems are family-based, rather than all centred in Maureen.

Within social work discourse, such an assessment has a sound basis in the theory of family therapy (e.g., Barker 1986), but the likelihood of the officer being able, in practice, to intervene in this family in the way she would have liked was remote, for two reasons. First, the ideology of the family still succeeds in holding the working-class mother responsible for any chaos which surrounds her:

> Maureen *is* chaotic [and] it does tend to generate chaos around her. Because it's the *woman* in that situation, it has far more impact on the family at large than if it was a man...Perhaps it's because the woman is the one who is always cast as the one who *should* do the coping and the managing and the looking after of the children. When men become ill, they become almost like another child for the woman to cope with, but the man doesn't seem to cope very well when it's the woman who is ill. It's like a cultural [thing] – with that particular generation – Women's Lib had no impact at all.

119

Second, both the psychiatrist and the social workers involved accepted, and thus reinforced, an assessment of the situation in which Maureen was identified as *the* problem:

> Social Services labelled her as a 'bad mother'; the psychiatrist just sees her as 'the patient'; husband just sees her as ' failed wife and mother' – nobody has actually spoken to Maureen as a woman, as a person in her own right.

The demand for the woman in a family to be the one responsible for bringing about change was also illustrated by a probation officer who was supervising both a husband and wife on probation. It was clear that his expectations of what could be achieved in work with the two clients varied greatly. His overall aim in the case was to improve communication between the couple but the focus was primarily on the wife:

> I've got her practising telling him specifically where she is going and talking to him about it when she comes back...He is more reporting as a probationer. He comes in and we play a game of pool or something like that.

> (Probation Officer 11)

Mary Eaton (1985) found that when probation officers were preparing social inquiry reports on men, they used home visits to meet and assess significant others (usually women) in the men's lives, whereas such visits in the cases of women were used to see what kind of home they maintained. Probation officers are also more keen to involve the female partners of men under supervision than the male partners of women. Implicit in this practice is the assumption that it is women who should influence and bring about change in relationships. A probation officer working at a day centre, whose clientele (as with all day centres) was predominantly male, told me:

> We are also attracting wives...or girlfriends of men who are clients. Some females [here] are not clients and are as near to volunteers as possible.

> (Probation Officer 12)

By the term 'volunteers' he was referring to the Service 'voluntary associates' who befriend clients and assist in other ways without payment. The use of the term in this context, however, seems somewhat ironic, given the level of choice which these women probably had within those relationships. The nature of that relationship was also heavily circumscribed. The 'volunteer' might very easily be reconstructed as the 'whore' if she overstepped the bounds of correct behaviour in this male domain, as the officer continued to explain:

> They may have a boyfriend who is at the Centre...that
> boyfriend may change from week to week, but they will tend to
> relate to a particular man. One or two of the women will tend
> to relate to a number of men. We've had suspicions, for
> example, about the activities of one of our females...about
> using us as a sort of picking up spot.

So, in order to be welcomed as a respectable influence at the centre, a woman must be seen to be attached to one particular man at any one time – almost, it seems, to be identified as 'someone's property' rather than 'lost property', since the latter becomes a threat to the good order and smooth running of the establishment.

When such relationships founder, it is again often the woman who is blamed. She is seen as exploiting the relationship for her own ends – as seducing/manipulating the gullible, vulnerable man. Probation Officer 13 described one of his female clients thus:

> Last year, through relationships with men, she went to the
> south of France and Holland, and she goes away for weekends.
> When there is somebody there showing interest in her and
> she's provided with money and support she can be quite
> presentable and she's quite a live wire.

To which one is tempted to reply, 'Aren't we all?' But the probation officer continues:

> Much of her life is based on deception...and she's certainly one
> of the most untruthful people I've ever met. And because she is
> so unreliable in what she says, she doesn't form relationships
> that last. She tends to abuse friendships. So we keep going
> round in cycles – she gets a friendship, she abuses it, she loses
> it, and she's down to rock bottom again.

The 'rooting' of largely unemployed, working-class women in relationships thus produces a paradoxical 'reality' in which:

1) They are expected to be 'providers' for their families but are denied the material resources with which to provide in a socially and legally approved manner.

2) They are held responsible for any dysfunction within their families and also for bringing about positive change in those families. This means that, while they suffer the stigma of being the 'identified patient' (or 'client'), they are not allowed to enjoy the 'benefits' of being ill.

3) While they are expected to be stabilizing influences on their wayward male partners, any attempt to reap satisfaction for themselves from these relationships is interpreted as 'abuse' of the relationship.

Probation officers are not unaware of these paradoxes, but find themselves powerless to offer alternative definitions of 'reality'. Since, in order to act as probation officers, they have first to define a situation within their own professional discourse, they often need to categorize (describe) their women clients in stereotypical ways. Probation Officer 14 summarizes the predicament in describing her own attempt to 'make sense' of one woman client:

> The choices are either to see her as a good woman, caring for her family but suffering from psychological disorder which causes lapses into anti-social behaviour, or, bluntly, to see her as a liar and a thief, who attempts to con her way out of difficult situations. The truth is, no doubt, in the grey area between.

Within the confines of such tensions, probation officers see themselves as offering what support, advice, and befriending they can, often using their limited time and material resources in imaginative and caring ways. Time after time they recounted situations where they felt they had gone beyond what was strictly required of them professionally to provide help for these women, or to try and introduce some interest and variety into their seemingly mundane and unrewarding lives. Time after time, however, they felt their attempts had been thwarted – partly by lack of co-operation from other professionals, but very often by the apparent indifference of the women themselves and/or the intractable nature of their problems. Probation Officer 15 told me in desperation about one woman:

> I feel I've had to wash my hands of her – I used to go twice a week.

The relentlessness of this level of demand, with little evidence of discernible progress, was but one of the frustrations which probation officers experienced in working with 'nondescript' women and these frustrations will now be considered in more depth.

CONTRACT AVOIDANCE – LOSING MODES?

The feelings of most officers seemed to be summed up in this comment by Probation Officer 13:

> The demands have been considerable and the input has been high – the rewards so far not very great.

While it is undoubtedly true that officers could identify many male clients of whom this could also be said, the additional frustration in working with women is the even greater rarity of 'breach' proceedings consequent to non-compliance with the conditions of supervision. Only one officer could recall taking breach proceedings against a woman and that was in an extreme situation:

> The reason the order was breached was that she refused to come in – entirely.
>
> (Probation Officer 3)

Officers tend to feel more powerless in relation to female clients:

> With women I never feel I have as much authority. Men seem to think, 'If I don't report, I could go to prison', whereas women realize that courts don't like sending them to prison. I think they pick that up, don't they?
>
> (Probation Officer 16)

Such a comment also illustrates the ambivalence felt by many probation officers about the degree of agency which can be imputed to women in their contract avoidance. Here, as in many other remarks, officers imply that the women deliberately and consciously (even if furtively) refuse to fulfil the obligations they undertook in court. In this, they reflected all those discourses within which women are constructed as being more devious than men. The manner of the delivery of these remarks was, however, frequently heavily ironic, in the sense that, whilst officers often felt that such behaviour was deliberate, they also recognized that it was their own frustration that had given them a sense of persecution and that the choice of response to supervision available to the women was often extremely limited.

The mechanisms whereby these women avoided the gender contract implicit in supervision were often ultimately self-defeating in that they failed to produce any sense of satisfaction or achievement for either the women or those who sought to help them. Such mechanisms could be described as 'defences of the weak' (Mathiesen 1972) and identified as mechanisms of:

a) elusiveness;
b) demand;
c) deviousness;
d) refusal.

Elusiveness – like a butterfly

The commonest complaint about women on probation was their inability/refusal to keep appointments. The following comments were typical:

I have difficulty getting them to report.
The majority I have to visit at home – I'd never get them in.

(Probation Officer 16)

She's unreliable, doesn't keep appointments and shows disinterest [sic].

(Probation Officer 13)

I talked to her basically about what probation was...to see if she'd be willing to come in. She made it a joke – 'Oh, don't you have to come here?'

(Probation Officer 3)

But home visiting had its problems as well. Probation Officer 7 talked about a voluntary associate who called 'religiously' every week on one young woman and her cohabitee:

> They know what time she's coming – and they go out!

Another of her female clients 'loved' her to visit but:

> She has her daughters visiting her on a Tuesday which is the day I visit. She did say she would change their visiting day, but never has and I don't know how much it is a protection.

> (Probation Officer 7)

This officer felt that the woman concerned was very unhappy but was fearful of discussing this openly with the officer and was using her daughters' visits to avoid becoming too involved in a relationship where self-disclosure was expected.

But elusiveness consists of more than mere physical avoidance of contact. Many probation officers became frustrated by the women's failure to tell them things which the officers considered to be important to discuss. For example, Probation Officer 7 told me how Pauline had

> shoplifted, been arrested and taken to the police station, went home in an absolutely distraught state, rang the Samaritans, told them about me but couldn't ring me.

This inability/refusal to engage in what was seen to be appropriate self-disclosure or confession (without which officers felt impotent to offer help within the discourses available to them) was one of the modes of behaviour which was categorized as 'not responding' to supervision. The following comments were typical:

> She doesn't respond.

> (Probation Officer 7)

> I really don't know where I am with this girl.

> (Probation Officer 9)

> I'm hardly able to have any influence on her life because she's like a butterfly.

> (Probation Officer 13)

In these situations, probation officers feel that the women 'go through the motions' of adhering to the conditions of their probation orders but lack commitment to changing their behaviour or attitudes. Evidence for this is seen to exist in the apparent readiness of the women to use family responsibilities as excuses for non-engagement – or mutedness. Beryl was conveniently being visited by her daughters every time her probation officer called; Jackie was accused by her officer of being 'not beyond using Zoe [her baby daughter] as an excuse for going home' and thus failing to co-operate fully with the treatment at the Special Treatment Unit. Probation Officer 16 described another young woman who 'seems to have a lot of insight into herself' but who, it was found on further examination, was simply repeating things that her mother had said to her:

> I don't think she has any of her own self-identity. She seems to have the identity that's given to her by other people. When I hear her talking, I think, 'That's her mum', because I know her mum and I know the way she speaks, and she's just repeating 'parrot' what her mum says.

The absence of 'self-identity' among the women was another feature of their 'rootedness' and their 'mutedness'. The women appeared to be defined – and to define themselves – in relation to other people and how they believed that other people viewed them:

> She is trying to find her own identity, but can't. She's struggling because she's got these conflicting things all the time.

(Probation Officer 16)

Given 'these conflicting things', it is perhaps not surprising that the women sometimes seemed indecisive. Jackie's inability/refusal to make up her mind about reconciling (or not) with her imprisoned husband led her probation officer (3) to declare in exasperation:

> I don't think she really knows what she wants.

The effect of this indecisiveness and lack of 'self-identity' was to leave probation officers feeling that they could never do any 'preventive' work with women. They rarely reached a stage where they felt that the women were able to anticipate problems or develop reliable coping strategies which might help to forestall crises:

> She's extremely mixed up and it's difficult to find a plan of action for her. You're always working from crisis to crisis.
>
> (Probation Officer 17)

> What you do at the point of crisis and how you resolve it doesn't lead her to understand how it developed and how it can be prevented.
>
> (Probation Officer 13)

Demands – like a baby

Having to respond constantly – and sometimes exclusively – at the point of crisis, without being able to help clients develop their own strategies for coping with and preventing future crises, in accordance with the accepted model of 'crisis intervention' work (e.g., O'Hagan 1986), is very wearing and actually creates a state of crisis in the worker him/herself. As was seen earlier, some workers eventually respond by withdrawing altogether because the level and nature of the demands become too great. Before that point is reached, probation officers seem to go through two phases of work with these women. First, they try 'to be around for the moment that she needs you' (Probation Officer 13).

They tolerate the physical avoidance and the lack of commitment, they persist in trying to build up a relationship of trust because they know that, sooner or later, the women will need someone to turn to:

> You often get men on probation without seeing any specific problem, but with women, it's chaos – they're almost all like that. But they tend to be not very forthcoming to get help....If things really get to a crisis [they] come in, so in that respect it is worthwhile.
>
> (Probation Officer 16)

This probation officer was implying that the 'Alternatives to

127

Custody' debate had resulted in men frequently being placed on probation because of their position on the 'tariff' (that is, because the nature of their offence or the number of their previous convictions placed them at risk of imprisonment). Women were still being placed on probation because they were viewed as being 'in need'. Consequently, a reluctance on the part of some women to demonstrate dependence on their probation officer was seen as of more significance than a similar reluctance on the part of men. Having nurtured that dependency, however, the officers then find that the demands of the women for an 'instant response' (Probation Officer 7) become difficult to control:

> If I'm not available she's very hurt and upset – very angry because [she feels] I *should* be there....She's like a baby – wants a feed, cries and demands it *now* – and that's not reality.
>
> (Probation Officer 7)

Once again, the issue of who has the right/power to define 'reality' intrudes. This officer felt that she was fortunate in that Pauline was viewed as 'a good person to work with, very intelligent and you can reason things through with her'. Most officers did not feel they could say this of the women they worked with – and even this officer was uncertain about the extent to which this 'insight' actually resulted in changed behaviour:

> She still hasn't got the answers as to why she shoplifts but she feels she's getting a bigger understanding of herself.

And, since probation orders are time-limited, there comes a point when the dependency has to cease. The stage of 'trying to wean her off' (Probation Officer 1) (the mamillary metaphor again) requires a redefinition of the problem of elusiveness:

> I'm *spacing* the contact a bit more and trying to give her lots of encouragement and pats on the back.
>
> (Probation Officer 1)

But there is a further frustration in working with nondescript women which exacerbates both their elusiveness and their demands. That further frustration arises from a feeling among probation officers that these women, far from being hapless victims, are rather 'stubborn and devious' (Probation Officer 6).

Deviousness – men con, women manipulate

Probation officers frequently describe themselves as 'being manipulated' by their women clients. The comparable term used in relation to male clients is 'being conned' and most officers pride themselves on their ability to detect men who are 'trying it on' or not telling the truth. It is apparently more difficult to detect such behaviour in women because it appears to take the form of selective truth telling, rather than outright 'lying'. Women, one is given to understand, are particularly adept at representing the truth in ways which compel workers to act against their better judgement. The technique employed appears to be one of saying what the worker wants to hear (conceding a point, agreeing with an argument, expressing gratitude, promising to change, etc.) but making those concessions conditional on securing certain responses from the worker. While all relationships are, to some degree, marked by manipulation, the dissonance and consequent frustration provoked in probation officers by nondescript women is due to their ability, despite being 'chaotic' and 'inadequate', to exploit the contradictions in the gender contract. Probation officers know that official discourse obliges them to buttress any desire on the part of these women to undertake approbated feminine roles, however passively or apparently disingenuously that desire is expressed. Challenging such expressions would involve the officer in accepting the woman's self-defined reality and openly acknowledging the inadequacies of existing definitions. The only alternative is to reconstruct such women as essentially manipulative – and therefore dismissable. The following remarks from a probation officer responsible for placing clients in Community Service projects illustrates the point:

> She was stroppy in the initial interview, telling us what she was
> and wasn't going to do and we got trapped into going along with
> it. She's manipulated us – her offences were 'false pretences'!
>
> (Probation Officer 17)

Because many women commit offences defined as acts of 'deception', there is an assumption that the women themselves are deceptive. Constructing women as always and already deceptive (cf. Pollak 1950) then makes it impossible for officers either to define reality in relation to these women or to accept their own definitions of reality. Thus, they remain forever unknowable. The consequence of this for officers was that, even when they were concerned about particular aspects of their clients' lives, they did not feel able to address these openly because they felt they could not assume that the women were being truthful. Three examples illustrate this. Probation Officer 7 was concerned that one woman client was engaging in prostitution. She described the woman as:

> *Rather an unknown quantity.* Lives in a flat on her own and is the subject of much neighbourhood gossip and accusation about having men up there. I suspect there's some truth in it, but of course she denies it. So I can never work with her on that one.

Probation Officer 6 was concerned that one of her clients was anorexic:

> I've done what I can but she's quite stubborn and devious – that's the wrong word. I don't mean evil – but she will cover up when she's not eating. She'll say, 'I'm eating more than I was' – which means she's not!

Probation Officer 9 had just received a letter from a woman client, saying that she had been sexually abused by her father, but the officer was unsure how to respond:

> Gillian is very attention-seeking...you can never tell whether she's telling the truth or not.

This seems particularly ironic when there is now a public campaign to encourage women to bring such abuse to the attention of the authorities.

Perhaps the most frustrating aspect of this perceived deviousness was the unpredictable moodiness of the women, which seemed to make any notion of planning meaningless and often served to sabotage attempts at co-operation between agencies working with the same woman:

> One minute she's all lovey dovey and the next minute she's up in arms slating everybody – she doesn't like the social worker, she doesn't like you – and this is how it goes.
>
> (Probation Officer 4)

> Sandra is a manipulative lady who plays off one agency against another. Caution and discretion are needed in dealing with her.

(Probation Officer 18)

Such 'playing off' of workers and agencies against each other may be seen as an example of the nondescript woman's ability to exploit the often contradictory interests which, as has been seen, these agencies have in her.

Deviousness was seen as a mechanism requiring a greater degree of agency than either elusiveness or making demands. Manipulative women were viewed as being quite powerful and their behaviour provoked anger amongst officers rather than understanding. Feeling used or exploited by the women, probation officers either became wary of making any sort of commitment to, or on behalf of, these women, or they adopted what might be termed a 'mother superior' stance, in which they regarded the women as children needing firm but loving handling. Either way, the women's behaviour was stripped of any meaning it might have in relation to the inappropriateness of the discourses within which the probation officers were struggling to assess them.

Refusal

Defiance, assertiveness, decisiveness were not common characteristics of nondescript women, but one or two examples were given by probation officers of women who appeared to reject openly the help that was offered to them. Jackie, as has been seen, nearly lost her chance of a probation order when she (albeit apparently jokingly) refused to agree to attend office appointments. Probation Officer 19 had gone to a great deal of trouble to persuade a fine default court to reduce one of his clients' fine and compensation order, only to find the woman far from grateful:

> I've never known compensation costs be squashed like that – absolutely amazing. She came out...with £20 odd (to pay) at a pound a week – and she objected!

Probation Officer 20 had undertaken the even more time-

131

consuming job of finding a choice of no less than three alternatives which *he* saw as solutions to a client's accommodation problems, including a place in a probation hostel:

> I wanted her to go to the hostel but she refused all three [alternatives]. She said to the magistrates, 'Please send me to prison'. After an adjournment, they sent her to prison! She got a six-month sentence, during which time she lost two months' remission for bad behaviour – throwing plates and hitting other women, and generally being disruptive.

Probation officers were frequently at a loss to understand such self-defeating behaviour yet, as O'Dwyer (O'Dwyer and Carlen 1985) has suggested, the line between surviving and failing to survive in situations of oppression is a very narrow one. These women were engaging in the emotional/social equivalent of 'cutting up'. Unable to 'hit back' at the system, they internalized their responses to its pains and tensions and self-mutilated in an attempt to remain independent of others' inroads upon them. Such behaviour may well be interpreted within the rhetoric of 'Alternatives to Custody' as demonstrating a lack of motivation or commitment to making 'constructive' use of the opportunity of a probation order. What is frequently misunderstood is that what is being avoided is not so much the probation contract as the gender contract and the fear that the former is bound to involve the latter. What is also frequently overestimated is the degree of choice which women have about alternative strategies both for avoiding crime and for negotiating with courts about their treatment. Poverty, isolation, and lack of self-esteem do not create conditions conducive to the negotiation of the rational, fair, and acceptable contract implied by the 'non-treatment paradigm' of probation practice.

CONCLUSION

Probation officers recognize that many of the women they work with cannot be labelled or defined within the discourses of femininity which constitute the gender contract. Nevertheless, such women are 'rooted in relationships' and trapped by the contradictory effects of that 'rootedness'. In their endeavours to defy description and avoid the gender contract, nondescript women employ mechanisms which are interpreted by probation officers as elusiveness, demands, deviousness, and (though rarely) refusal. These mechanisms are regarded by probation officers as being self-defeating or losing modes of behaviour which lead officers to experience feelings of frustration and powerlessness. Similar feelings are engendered in probation officers by solicitors, psychiatrists, social workers, and magistrates who, they feel, not only fail to appreciate the restricted range of legitimate responses available to working-class, poor women, but who, through their own discursively circumscribed practices, actually restrict even further the choices available to these women. Despite these frustrations, it is possible for probation officers to experience a sense of achievement when, in the absence of any alternative provision, the contradictions of the gender contract are exploited to the benefit of women clients or when some women are empowered to find non-self-destructive solutions to the gender contract for themselves. It is to the discovery of these 'winning modes' that the next chapter addresses itself.[1]

Chapter Eight

LISTENING TO WOMEN – A FOOTNOTE?

Thirteen women were identified to me by their probation officers as 'troublesome' women, who might, nevertheless, be prepared to discuss with me their experiences of the criminal justice system. Of these, two (Jean and Linda) refused to be interviewed. Jean, according to her probation officer, was 'going through a crisis' and was preoccupied, while Linda was apparently not interested in discussing her experiences. Two other women (Susan and Kathy) both agreed to be interviewed but each failed to keep two appointments made with me. Mention has already been made of the trap in which these women are caught, whereby they are rendered incapable of either refusing or fulfilling the contract which is offered to them in the name of help. The mechanisms of resistance which are available to them are those which inevitably invoke from their would-be helpers moral judgements about 'unreliability', 'manipulativeness', and 'deceitfulness'. For those would-be helpers to consider any other, less positivistic explanation for the women's behaviour would threaten the 'taken-for-grantedness' of existing social relations. Failure to keep appointments and general elusiveness characterized many of the women who were discussed with me by their probation officers. Few of them could be accused of deliberately failing to keep in touch (which would constitute a breach of the conditions of a probation order) but time and time again, women would present reasons/excuses for being unable to keep office appointments (children's illnesses, lack of bus fares, repair men/Social Security visitors expected, etc.) yet would also find themselves unexpectedly called out of their homes when the officer had arranged to call on them. Even probation officers who laid on transport to bring women to women's groups or clubs run at their offices expressed frustration at the numerous abortive journeys made by volunteers or ancillary workers to women who were 'out' or whose children were suddenly and conveniently 'poorly'. These women, like Victoire Rivière (Foucault 1975), were the everlasting cancellers of contracts. Their potency lay in their ability to agree to, yet to fail to honour, even the simplest contracts about times and places of physical meetings. By presenting constantly moving targets, such women unwittingly succeeded in outwitting officials and evading assessment, classification, and control. For some women, their children – and their social workers, the consequences of such elusiveness can be tragic, especially when there is real concern for the welfare of children (cf. the Jasmine Beckford case, London Borough of Brent 1985). But while women remain distrustful of those in authority who are directed to 'help' them and, furthermore, feel powerless to influence the nature of that help, they will continue to put themselves literally 'beyond help' and 'out of reach' by simply avoiding contact.

Nine women, therefore, agreed to be interviewed and two more, as previously mentioned, were interviewed under different circumstances (Fiona and Jackie). In the interviews they talked about their law-breaking, their personal circumstances, their attitudes to courts, solicitors, psychiatrists, probation officers, social workers – and to themselves. Common themes emerged from their stories – loneliness, fear, low self-esteem, bewilderment, suppressed anger, and, above all, a sense of not being listened to, heard, or understood. But there were differences and contradictions, too. Some felt they had been sentenced harshly, but were still appreciative of the help they had received from individual professionals. Others felt they had been dealt with leniently, despite denying criminal intention or *mens rea*, in its strict judicial sense.

LAW-BREAKING/DEVIANCE – THE CONSTRUCTION OF (WO)MEN'S REA

With the exception of Carol ('I'm a shoplifter'), the women did not see themselves as 'real' criminals. They felt that what they had done either was not really criminal, or was a kind of 'compulsion', or had been done out of economic necessity. In its strict judicial sense, they denied criminal intention.

> I've not done anything really terrible. It was just a fight that got blown up into something big. I was done for conspiracy. I only drove the car. There was one other girl and five boys.
>
> (Fiona)

> On the form it says, 'with intent to deprive so-and-so of the aforesaid jar of coffee...' and it didn't seem – well, I'd been in hospital.
>
> (Ivy)

> I defrauded my husband of his supplementary benefit – I cashed his Giro....I went to the police station myself to own up – they didn't find out...I agreed to probation, but I didn't think it would be two years.
>
> (Eileen)

> It was for food for my children – it wasn't stupid things like cigarettes or drink or toys.
>
> (Veronica)

> I sort of get this feeling that I've *got* to get something off the shelves – and when I've done it and got out of the shop, I think it's great.
>
> (Janet)

> One day my little girl...showed me under her mattress – £86. She said it belonged to a boy – he wanted her to look after it. He'd said I could borrow £30...so I borrowed it....The police came and I explained, but they said I should have reported it.
>
> (Maureen)

> I didn't really think I'd done anything wrong.
>
> (Gwen)

Even Carol was indignant about the latest offence with which she had been charged, although she was pessimistic about her chances of acquittal:

> Carol: I'm not guilty, I didn't do it, yet I'll probably get found guilty because of my record. They look at your record and they'll say 'I don't believe she didn't do something like that'.
>
> AW: But they're not supposed to know your record until you're found guilty.
>
> Carol: Aye, well that is true, but the judge knows me.

Despite their denials of guilt, all of the women, like Carol, eventually resigned themselves to being 'found guilty', partly because of their low self-esteem and generalized sense of guilt about being a woman and thus 'always and already' failing, but partly as a result of being treated as though they were always and already guilty. Pauline illustrates the former:

> I expected a lot worse and, quite honestly, I felt I deserved a lot worse – I still do....I still feel that I haven't been punished – yet nobody else seems to.

Fiona, Ivy, and Gwen illustrate the latter:

> At court I stood between two prison officers thinking 'I'm really ever such a nice person – I shouldn't be here.' In my statement, I signed for a lot of things I didn't say because I was afraid. You say things, but not in the way they put it over in court – out of context.
>
> (Fiona – changed plea during trial)

> They're only doing their job – the prosecuting counsel – he's got to make it hard, hasn't he? And I did do wrong.
>
> (Ivy – defended herself, but was found guilty)

> When I was in the van, he told them over the microphone that I was a prisoner. I said to him, 'I'm not a prisoner'. Well, I wasn't at the time – or was I? He said, 'We've now got the prisoner' and that upset me.
>
> (Gwen – arrested after throwing a brick through her own house window)

Uncertainty about appropriate pleading was not always alleviated by solicitors and the women expressed mixed feelings about the role of solicitors in court. None of the women saw themselves as 'engaging the services' of solicitors or 'giving instructions' nor did they feel in any way in control of their relationship with their solicitor. Some, though, did express gratitude for their solicitor's efforts:

> I think that the solicitor does a lot – it's the way he puts your case over....I think that really makes a difference...because you can tell a story or explain things different ways and it comes out differently.
>
> (Pauline)

> I mean really it's not up to them – they try their best....He was very good. I thought I'd go down....
>
> (Veronica)

But even Veronica did not seem to feel very much in control of the relationship, especially once her solicitor had engaged a barrister for the case:

> I didn't really have much to say to him. He just said, 'Don't worry'. He didn't say one thing or the other.

This inability to express oneself to a solicitor or barrister featured in other women's accounts:

> He got a barrister from London but he didn't give me any advice about the plea. The trial went on for five days and at the end I changed my plea to guilty.
>
> (Fiona)

> I couldn't talk to him like I'm talking to you now. I couldn't fight for myself. I couldn't defend myself. I couldn't give him enough evidence to go on to defend me.
>
> (Maureen)

Maureen perceived her encounter with her solicitor as something of an ordeal – as one more situation in which she was required to justify herself and her actions. Like most of the women, she felt herself to be insufficiently articulate to benefit from this 'right' to be represented. The whole point of representation – namely, the opportunity to compensate for nervousness, ignorance, and inarticulacy – was lost on these women, thus providing an excellent example of the 'technology of muting'. Women defendants are given a formal right to a space where they can tell their story in their own words to someone who can then reconstruct it in language which is acceptable to the court. Yet the experience of most women is that they must already have structured their tale in a way which is acceptable to the court. Yet again, as with their encounters with psychiatrists, working class women experience the double oppression of both gender and class discrimination in their dealings with white, middle-class, professional men. Carol – perhaps the most articulate of the women (but also the only black woman, which may or may not have been significant) – challenged her solicitor by playing according to the stated rules of the game – and suffered the consequences:

> I don't care, I just talk to them....I tell them the truth and own up if I've done it. Then they advise me to plead guilty or not guilty. But he always says with my record I'll get sent down. I don't think they should do that. I think they should fight for you.

Two of the women did not have solicitors in court. Gwen, despite her contact with a probation officer, appeared unaware of her right to representation:

> I think if you've never been in trouble before, you don't know, do you?

She did, in fact, approach a solicitor after she had been sentenced to probation with a condition of in-patient psychiatric treatment. Not surprisingly, she did not get much satisfaction at that stage:

> I went to a solicitor to see if he could get me off the probation so that I could get out of the hospital but he said there wasn't much they could do because they couldn't do anything but put me in hospital.

Ivy was the one woman who had decided to defend herself, although her reasons for doing so were not entirely clear:

> AW: Why did you not want a solicitor?
> Ivy: I don't know really....
> AW: Was it a question of thinking you would have to pay?

Ivy: Yes, I suppose it was....My doctor did write a letter, which I can't understand was not read out prior to my being sentenced. I feel that that should perhaps have been taken into account....

Ivy believed that her medical condition rendered her 'morally' innocent of the offence with which she was charged but she seemed unable to distinguish between its legal status as a defence or as mitigation. Consequently, she had not known when to introduce her doctor's letter into her evidence and the result was that it had been overlooked. Perhaps more ironically, Ivy's competence in defending herself later had negated her claim to having been confused at the time of the alleged offence. Her failure to remain mute had been her downfall. In the end, she admitted reluctantly:

Maybe I should have had a solicitor but we had one for that other do and it never got us anywhere.

Many of these women's experiences are common to all defendants (cf. Carlen 1976). There is, however, a specific gender dimension to their experiences which is characterized by

a) *the particular social disgrace of being a criminal woman:*

It's far less acceptable for a woman to commit a crime. A man sometimes gets a boost from it – a woman loses any respect she had once people know she's got a record.

(Fiona)

b) *the sense of guilt and low self-esteem which many women have about themselves as women:*

I'm inclined to blame myself and that has a lot to do with my state now – I'm blaming myself for being a failure.

(Ivy)

c) *the apparent difficulty which many women have in communicating* what they really want to say (if indeed they know what they really want to say) to men in positions of authority – in this case, to solicitors and barristers. This apparent difficulty may be not so much a failure on the part of women to articulate their needs, as a failure on the part of men in authority to listen to the particular

140

mode of expression in which those needs are being communicated.

d) *the particular requirement that women who break the law* must compensate for their 'unfeminine' criminal behaviour by presenting themselves as domesticated, sexually passive, and constitutionally fragile.

Before turning to this last requirement and examining these women's own accounts of their domesticity, sexuality, and pathology, it is important to note all the aspects of the gender dimension which have been outlined have a class bias in their effects. Educated and financially independent women, although still experiencing the stigma of criminality, have more options in the ways that they choose to re-present themselves or allow themselves to be re-presented. They may still suffer from a 'sense of guilt' and 'low self-esteem' but they have the articulacy and the finances to escape the most confining of stereotypical descriptions. Working-class women have to devise more devious escape-routes.

DOMESTICITY

Motherhood

Undoubtedly and according to all concerned the most important relationships for those women who were mothers were those with their children. Whether or not their children were in their care, their attitudes towards them were profoundly and inextricably bound up with their attitudes to their law-breaking. On the one hand, children were cited by the women as both the cause of and the justification for criminal activity. On the other hand, they were seen by them as exerting a restraining influence both on the women themselves and on those sentencing them.

Committing crime *for* the children

The desire to provide material goods, which they could not otherwise afford, for their children motivated most of the shoplifters. Some saw themselves stealing 'essentials'; others saw their activity as a way of providing 'extras':

It was food for my children. It wasn't stupid things like
cigarettes or drinks or toys – you know, rubbish.

(Veronica)

I like to keep my kids nice and I like to have a nice house.

(Carol)

It was Jane's birthday and I'd gone to town to buy some candles
for her cake, and it started that I picked up something in
Woolworth's and I was thinking 'I'd like to buy this....I can take
it and nobody will know, and I can give it to her, although I
can't afford it.' So I did, and then it just snowballed.

(Pauline)

The desire to be the stereotypically good mother and provider
had led some of the women into activity which could ultimately
deprive them of the very people they sought to provide for.

Committing crime *because of* the children

For some of the women, however, the influence of their children
on their law-breaking was more complex. Gwen's offence, for
example, seems to have been committed at least in part from a
sense of frustration and desperation about the difficulties she was
experiencing in maintaining contact with her daughter in Care:

AW: Can you remember why you put the bricks through the
        windows?
Gwen: It was everything all muddled up. It was my neighbours
        and because I hadn't got my daughter.

For Maureen, her children and their behaviour, together with her
husband's behaviour, constituted the chaotic domestic environment
from which she could escape only into crime or mental illness:

I went into the living room and the table was full...and I'd just
put the baby down and I wanted to rest and everybody was just
gawping at the television. So I walked in and tipped the table
up and said, 'You can sodding well clean this lot up between
you – I'm not the slave here.'

Feeling unsupported and unappreciated featured in both
Maureen and Ivy's accounts. Maureen's strongest criticism was
reserved for her daughter:

My eldest son will...go out and buy me an extra bag of coal. He
looks after me, he appreciates what I'm doing for him. But my

daughter – she thinks I only want her for her money!
Sometimes I feel like punching her in the face, 'cos I'm very
highly strung.

Ivy had two daughters and a son, all of whom had left home –
as had her husband. She disliked her son's girlfriend and blamed
herself for her son's departure from home at the age of 28:

> I find that I'm obsessed with losing my son – I felt I had driven
> him away

She spoke movingly of the increasing loneliness she felt as her
family gradually left her:

> At night – you've been used to having five people there, then
> it's four, then it's three, and now it's me. I find it very hard to
> live alone. Not so much in the day, but at night. I miss the key
> coming and the voices.

It had been suggested to me by some probation officers that
women often failed to face up to the 'reality' of their law-
breaking and its consequences. A probation officer working in a
women's prison, however, argued that, for many of the women
he met, providing for their families *was* reality. Even when those
families had disintegrated, the women continued to define
themselves in relation to them and to be, in his words, 'rooted in
relationships'.

The effect of crime *on* the children

Only Carol spoke of her criminal activity having any direct effect
on her children:

> Carol: It's embarrassing. You don't like them to know. I mean,
> they know what I'm doing, but I wouldn't take them
> out and let them see that I'm doing it.
> AW: Have any of them ever been in trouble?
> Carol: Joe was in trouble once – he stole some sweets.
> AW: What happened to him?
> Carol: Nothing – he was too young. But I've told them, if they
> ever do anything I'll get the police. There's one thief in
> the house and that's enough. They don't need to do
> anything because I'm doing it for them.

Although Carol felt some 'embarrassment' about her children's knowledge of her activity, one could also sense that she took pride in sacrificing her own reputation for her children's well-being. Her son's foray into crime concerned her not so much because she felt she might be setting him a bad example but because it represented 'ingratitude' and a lack of appreciation of her as a good mother and provider.

For most of the women, however, their greatest fear was that of losing their children as a result of their criminal activity. Carol's attitude was thus not typical. She regarded imprisonment as an occupational hazard and even as a 'holiday' – 'because it's a break away from the kids'. Her children went into Care while she was in prison and visited her regularly. She had no fears that they might not be returned to her:

> I put them in myself and they couldn't take them off me. I don't ill-treat them and they get everything they want.

Maureen had been far less confident when she had gone to prison:

> It says 'voluntary' on the papers but...they watch them and if they think they need 'Care and Protection', you don't get them back. I kept thinking, 'I won't get her back'. I was more worried over losing my child than anything.

Eileen feared that her children would be taken into Care when she went to court because:

> My husband's in prison...I've had two broken marriages.

She had not responded previously to help offered by her probation officer or psychiatrist:

> Eileen: I didn't want any help. It's only been since [court] that I've wanted anybody to help me.
> AW: Did you think that your children were going to go away?
> Eileen: Yes, in [court] I did – and since then I'll sit and listen.

Jackie had received a similar message:

> The magistrate said 'We want you to sort yourself out – we're thinking of your child – we don't want to see you here again.'

144

As an inmate of a Special Treatment Unit, Jackie was separated from her daughter during the week but allowed to go home at weekends. She viewed the separation very much as punishment, rather than as the unavoidable consequence of receiving treatment in a hospital setting. She regarded her sentence as a kind of imprisonment, from which she could not resist the temptation to 'abscond':

> I don't want to stay here much longer. I miss my daughter terribly. I really love her and she loves me – she clings to me. That's why I ran off last week. You just sit here all day listening to records and I think of all the things I could be doing at home. I've got a nice home – I keep it really clean and tidy.

The notion that, by sitting and 'listening to records', she might be learning to be a better mother – when she could be keeping her home 'nice' – clearly struck her as faintly ridiculous.

Fear of losing their children dictated the attitude of these women to their local authority social workers. With the exception of Carol ('I need a shoulder to cry on – I'm not too old for that'), those who spoke about their social workers did so in fairly negative terms. Eileen summarized the general view:

> I fetched 'em [children] into the world and I didn't fetch 'em in for the Welfare to grab hold of 'em.

She admitted, reluctantly, that her present social worker was being quite helpful 'because they've just got a holiday granted for my children', but reiterated her general view:

> I always thought social workers were nasty people who all they wanted to do was take people's children into Care.

Gwen also experienced her previous social workers as unhelpful, condescending, authoritarian, and in a hurry:

> Social workers don't seem to be much help – that's why I lost my little girl...They give you the feeling that they're doing you a favour when they're helping you...They seem to show more authority to you. When you tell them your problem, they're in and out, and you're still there with your problem.

Like Eileen, Gwen was also more favourably disposed towards her current social worker because 'she explains things to me' and she had also arranged for Gwen to get out of the house to a weekly activities group.

As we shall see later in this chapter, the 'alleviation of loneliness' is one of the most important kinds of 'help' which these women seek and expect from their social workers and probation officers. It is also worth noting that, while probation officers were expected to use their authority and were not resented for doing so, social workers were given any credit by the women only when they produced specific 'goodies'. They were also more likely than probation officers to be attributed with 'enjoying' doing controlling things, like taking children away from home.

But although the women were fearful that their law-breaking might lead to their separation from their children and that they therefore needed, at the least, to pay lip-service to reforming themselves, they were also conscious that their status as mothers would influence sentences in their favour. Hilary Walker has demonstrated that attempts to blackmail sentencers emotionally can backfire disastrously (1985: 68), but Veronica was openly prepared to take that risk:

> They did ask who would look after [my son] if I went down. I said I didn't know – they'd have to have him put away in Care. That wasn't really true – my family wouldn't have let it go that far. But I played on that. You've got to play on something, haven't you?

Pauline was far less openly manipulative, but when I asked her why she felt she had been dealt with (by her own account) so sympathetically, she replied:

> Maybe it's the fact that I've got to support two children. Had I been a single girl, perhaps it might have been different. I don't know, but I think that would sway *me* if I was in their position.

Being a mother, then, was the most important feature of these women's lives and the loss of their children – whether physically, through care proceedings, or emotionally, through arguments or simply growing up – was the thing they feared most and which most threatened their respect for themselves as women.

Wifeliness

In contrast to the importance of children, husbands were

generally discussed in far less detail and the marital relationship described in fatalistic terms. By and large, the women appeared to expect their marriages to be unsatisfactory. The exception was Jackie, who remained optimistic about mending her marriage, although her romantic view of married life bore little relation to the reality of her situation, since her husband was in prison for assaulting her (cf. Carlen 1983: 36):

> I've sorted my problems out and so has he. I just want us to be dead happy together with the baby.

Two women had found their husbands less than supportive during their court proceedings:

> AW: Has your husband ever helped with your fines?
> Janet: No. When I had the TV licence fine, I had to keep going back to court.
>
> AW: Did your husband go to court with you?
> Ivy: No...I thought that was a bit mean of him, actually...I had to phone because I was getting in a state.

Only three of the women (Janet, Maureen, and Ann) were actually living with their husbands at the time of the interviews and two spoke of a lack of communication and understanding:

> AW: Did your husband object at all to your doing Community Service?
> Janet: He doesn't know.
> AW: Does he know you're on probation?
> Janet: Yes.
> AW: Is there any reason why you don't want him to know about Community Service?
> Janet: Well, we don't speak about a lot of things.

> People don't realize that men go through a change of life...If I didn't think on those lines, I'd have thought my marriage was breaking up and I'd be divorcing him. He doesn't take a bit of notice of me – I could be a cabbage in that house – and then just coming to me when he wants.
>
> (Maureen)

Despite a long history of marital disharmony, Maureen was still prepared to excuse her husband's behaviour as 'menopausal', although no such excuses seem to have been allowed for her behaviour.

Eileen also accepted her husband's behaviour – in this case, his violence – as a normal part of marriage, and she was very uncertain about whether she would eventually divorce her third husband, who was in prison at the time:

> Eileen: We've chopped and changed our minds that much over the past eight months. We've been apart twelve months – he's been in prison eight months. At the back of my mind is I know that if he comes home he'll hit me.
>
> AW: Do you think anyone will be able to help you with that when he comes out?
>
> Eileen: No, I'm going to take it. If he comes out and he feels better after hitting me, let him hit me. That's my attitude.

The tendency of women to blame themselves when their marriages fail was also illustrated in Ivy's account. Her husband left her and went to live with her best friend:

> Mainly perhaps it was because of my fault that he left...I can see now that perhaps I wasn't very tolerant of him.
>
> (Ivy)

Ivy had known about her husband's affair for some time ('he went out with this person three times a week') but felt guilty for criticizing him because she also 'had got a friend'. Nevertheless, it seemed that she had worked hard to ensure that her 'extra-marital' friendship did not interfere with her role in the home:

> That was a thing apart – my home and family were first.

Her husband, on the other hand, had been prepared – as she saw it – to sacrifice his family for his affair. Her anger towards him was not totally disguised but she had coped with her feelings largely by taking on board all the guilt and blame for the failure of the marriage – and had suffered the consequent loss of self-confidence:

> I used to have lots of confidence, which I don't have now. I rely on my family – I watch the clock until they come. This isn't *me*. I never knew the meaning of the word 'loneliness'.

Loss of confidence and self-esteem as a wife and mother were further exacerbated by the fear of 'neighbourliness' – the fear of having one's 'criminality' discovered by friends, neighbours, and relatives through the dreaded medium of the local paper:

> It was in the papers eight times – I had to cut it out. I got into more trouble because I wouldn't let anyone come to my home. The police kept ringing and telling me to go to the station – I couldn't say no.
>
> (Fiona)

> I don't want anyone to know what I'm doing because I know it will be in the papers and if Mum finds out it will break her heart.
>
> (Pauline)

AW: Was anything in the papers?
Ivy: I looked and I thought 'Good grief, I hope nothing is' – I didn't see anything.
AW: Have you had any comments from neighbours?
Ivy: I never told anyone.

AW: Was there anything in the local paper about it?
Janet: Yes. I've had lots of comments from neighbours – half of them don't speak to me. I lost my job over it.

SEXUALITY

Perhaps unsurprisingly, most of the women interviewed did not talk about their 'sexuality'. Perceiving criminal activity as an expression of a woman's sexuality is a pastime indulged in more by those who seek to classify, judge, and reform women than by those women themselves. As Heidensohn (1985: 93) observes, 'alongside the witch, the whore is the most potent image of female deviance', but, unlike mental illness, it is not an identity which women themselves are ready to accept in order to minimize their punishment.

Carol was quite clear on that, while shoplifting was an acceptable way to make money, prostitution was not:

> I could be a hustler, but I'm not giving my body away, so I steal.
> At least I've got some pride.

She was also very dismissive of those social workers and probation officers who had implied that her violent cohabitee might be meeting some psycho-sexual need in her:

> People say 'Get him out' but you can't just do that. I've been with him seven years – and he's violent. Did you read in the papers about a man raping a woman at knife-point? That was him – and he got off. That's what they call justice – he gets off and I get sent down for shoplifting £39.

Eileen insisted that accounts of her promiscuity were much exaggerated:

> I got involved with a man in September – and they said I was sleeping around.

Jackie was the only woman who admitted that she was a prostitute but she maintained her personal integrity by detaching herself emotionally from her clients and ensuring that she went 'only so far' with them (cf. McLeod 1982). As with Carol, 'pride' was an important criterion:

> I've never had intercourse. I only give 'hand-shakes' and do kinky things. I wouldn't give them my body or take anyone home. I've got my pride. It's just easy money.

For Jackie, prostitution was clearly preferable to other employment that might be available to her:

> I've had a couple of jobs, but I've never really needed work. I've always had 'Sugar Daddies'. I can get what I want out of men.

As an inmate of a Special Treatment Unit, Jackie's prostitution had been attributed to psychopathology (cf. Glover 1969). Her own account suggests that the explanation for her behaviour lay more in the realm of economics than emotions. She was not, however, unaffected by the attitudes of those close to her. Unlike McLeod's prostitutes (1982: 34) she had not been rejected by her family, nor had she distanced herself from their controls. Like the other women I spoke to, she was not easy to categorize. Her life was full of contradictions and paradoxes, as she struggled to make sense of economic disadvantage and physical and emotional abuse.

PATHOLOGY

Of the fifteen women, only two had no involvement with psychiatrists and even these women referred to their own feelings in 'psychiatric' terms, thus indicating the extent of the influence of images of pathology in relation to female law-breaking. Fiona spoke of the depression she experienced following her offence, the fear of her parents' discovering it by reading the papers, and the guilt she felt when her father died while the case was being processed. At the other end of the spectrum, the 'professional' shoplifter, Carol, spoke of her stealing activity as being almost a compulsion:

> It's just that I go into a shop and...if the woman goes away and leaves me, I've just got to take something...I just can't be trusted.

> (Carol)

She received little sympathy, however:

AW: Sometimes when women get into trouble, people say they must be sick...

Carol: They've never said that to me. My social worker says I just live too high above my means.

Among the 'already-labelled' women, however, there was a surprising reluctance to accept the 'sick role' (cf. Chesler 1974; Procek 1980). Ivy and Maureen had the longest histories of mental illness and both, it might be argued, had taken on a 'sick role' as a response to their powerlessness in the family (Messerschmidt 1987). Nevertheless, they both struggled against being defined as 'abnormal':

> I've woken up petrified at about 4.30 in the morning and taken Valium...I get very lonely inside, a feeling of unreality...a feeling of not quite being normal. [But] when I look at it in another respect, I think, 'you silly fool, you – you're the same as anyone else'.

> (Ivy)

> One day I ran out of tablets and I didn't bother to get any more, and I slept without better – more of a natural sleep. And

I went to the doctor and said, 'I don't want any more nerve tablets' and she said, 'You what? You've had no side effects?' and I said 'No'. I haven't taken them from that day to this. I mean, I'm very highly strung. The house – it gets me down...but now I don't let it get me that bad.

(Maureen)

Pauline had been diagnosed as a depressive and referred to a psycho-therapeutic group, which she enjoyed very much (I just trot along because I like going!'). Nevertheless, she made a clear distinction between herself and the other members of the group:

Pauline: Out of a group of about six of us, three would be depressives with something in common and there's the girl with a phobia, and then there's another girl who gets temper tantrums with her depression and then there's me...I try to understand how they feel but I can't really know what it's like.

AW: Would you describe yourself as having depression?

Pauline: No, I don't think I have depressions. I have times when I'm upset and worried...I feel rotten about everything but that's not the same thing.

The three women who had been classified as 'problem drinkers' (Jackie, Ann, and Veronica) all denied that their problems were either current or chronic. Jackie claimed to have been 'dry' for twelve weeks but did not envisage having to remain totally abstinent: 'I'm not a real alcoholic'. She calculated that alcohol was not problematic for her unless combined with Ativan (a tranquillizer), to which she had been – but was no longer – addicted. Ann's response was almost identical:

I used to have a drink problem, although it took me a long time to admit it.

She, too, had been addicted to Ativan but claimed she had not taken any drugs for two weeks. Veronica also claimed that her heavy drinking days were a thing of the past:

AW: What about the drink problem you said you had – do you still get that?

Veronica: Well occasionally – but not like I used to. I used to be drinking all the while...Then I just plucked up

courage one day and says, 'No more drink' – and I
went for about eighteen months.

These comments suggest that these women had learned that,
whether or not their drinking had actually diminished, denial of
a drink problem would not prevent intervention by professionals,
who regard such denial as a classic defence mechanism of
alcoholism. Rather than resist such intervention openly, they had
learned to accommodate the powerlessness of their gender/class
position (Messerschmidt 1987) by admitting the problem, but
only as a past feature of their lives. By such means they were
credited with having some insight into their problems but they
also succeeded in neatly side-stepping responsibility for change, if
they did not wish to change.

After years of such evasion and passive non-co-operation, such
women had succeeded in being defined as having 'personality
disorders, not amenable to treatment'. But what had been the
women's expectations and experiences of 'treatment'? On the
whole, there was a marked disparity between what women had
expected (or wanted) of psychiatry and how they experienced it. It
is not insignificant that the woman who had the happiest
experiences of 'treatment' (Pauline) was not receiving drug therapy.
Psychotherapy – the opportunity to talk about oneself – was what
most of the women expected from psychiatry. Those who could
identify that element in their treatment were markedly more
satisfied with their deal than those who could not. Jackie and Eileen,
both of whom had experienced the 'therapeutic community'
atmosphere of a Special Treatment Unit, had found 'treatment'
reasonably beneficial. By contrast, those who had experienced ECT,
drug therapy, or ludicrously brief, curt 'consultations' had found the
experience alienating, confusing, and humiliating. The experience
of Susan (a non-responder), recounted by her probation officer, is
typical of many women on probation with conditions of treatment:

> From her description of what is happening, she is asked if she
> is all right, is her family all right, is she managing to cope, fine
> thank you, I'll make another appointment. She goes for two
> minutes each time and she feels she has no confidence in the
> psychiatrist...She never knows who it is she's seen, but from
> what I can gather, it tends to vary a bit.
>
> (Probation Officer 6 on Susan)

153

A number of the women actually claimed that they felt worse after ECT and drug therapy than they had done before. Ivy had felt quite disorientated after ECT:

> I would never have electric shock treatment again – it does something to the brain. It's helpful perhaps at the time, but it blocks out great masses of things that have happened. But it doesn't block out the nasty parts – if you understand.
>
> People tend to think that when you come out of hospital that you're quite better, when in fact, that's not always the case – it takes time to adjust yourself. Looking back on it now – well it's horrific. You still get this confused state.

Veronica had been prescribed Valium, but she had felt they were 'no good':

> You were losing your days all the while – you didn't know what you was doing with them. You was asleep all the while. That's no good for you. So I just put them down the toilet one day, and I've never had them since.

Maureen, as we have seen, also decided to give up her tablets because she became horrified by her dependency on them:

> I sometimes got left without [tablets] and I'd cry and my eyes were red and I'd go down to the doctor and I was ashamed to be in that state. Then he'd give them me and I'd be all right. But it used to give me banging heads.

While she had been in prison, she had also experienced the humiliation (cf. Peckham 1985) of having to queue for her medication:

> In there I was on Valium, Tryptizol, Prochlorol, and tablets for me kidneys and me bowels. Three times a day – all that lot – can you imagine? In fact, they called me the 'drug squad' at the blooming clinic. *Although I didn't want it,* the doctor was giving me this and I felt terrible with girls standing behind me having two things and I was having five things at a time.
>
> (emphasis added)

Gwen was in hospital for three months, receiving Modecate injections which seemed to make her extremely lethargic. She had few visitors and became increasingly fearful of becoming institutionalized:

> When you don't have visitors it makes you worse because you're getting more into the routine of hospital.

The doctor had told her, she said, that the more active she kept, the more likely she would be to be discharged. But, she explained,

> I used to do a lot of sewing and things but I stopped doing it.
> He said, 'If you start doing your sewing and doing things you're more likely to be discharged.' But I got so that I couldn't do it – and I think that was the injections.

Eventually, in exasperation, she found the courage to walk out, and when I interviewed her several months later, declared that she felt 'much better' without the injections.

Women like Susan, Ivy, Maureen, and Gwen clearly experienced psychiatry more as control and punishment than as 'treatment'. Ann, in fact, said that she preferred prison to hospital. They were also very fearful of the power of their psychiatrists. As working-class women, they were doubly muted in their relationships with middle-class, professional men – by class and by gender. Susan's probation officer illustrates the problem:

PO 6: I've said, 'Why don't you tell him you think it's a waste of time?'

AW: That's a bit much to expect, isn't it?

PO 6: Well, not in those words! But I've suggested what she could say, but she won't, *because she'll avoid the problems....*

(emphasis added)

So it is the woman, yet again, who gets blamed.

But the psychiatrist's power – and the women's fear of it – was seen to extend beyond the hospital and the surgery – into a) the court and b) the home. The psychiatrist's expressed willingness to offer 'treatment' was seen as an important prerequisite for obtaining a lenient (i.e., non-custodial) sentence. As has been seen in the case of Kathy, even a charge of murder can result in a probation order if such an offer is forthcoming – even if it is never honoured (see also Allen 1987a). Conversely, a report from a psychiatrist declaring a defendant to be 'not mentally ill' or 'not amenable to treatment' is likely to render the defendant more liable to imprisonment than she might have been without a report at all. Veronica was very pessimistic after the psychiatrist had said he thought she was 'perfectly all right':

> Veronica: So that's when I thought I'd go down because I didn't have very good reports.
> AW: You hoped that he would say you needed treatment?
> Veronica: Yes, that's it – but he didn't. He was very nice – but, you know...he wasn't on my side.

Two of the women believed that it lay in their psychiatrists' power to remove their children from them – or return their children to them. Eileen's psychiatrist had made a rare domiciliary visit to observe her as a mother, in her 'natural' environment:

> Eileen: He came to the house just before Christmas – to see the children. He'd seen me in hospital as a patient, but he'd never seen me as a mother.
> AW: Do you think he was able to get a good impression of you at home?
> Eileen: Well, he's told me to keep my children – he's done a report.

Gwen's daughter had already been removed from her and she believed that her psychiatrist would block any attempt by her to get her daughter back:

> I was thinking of going to court, but I suppose Dr C only has to say *he* doesn't think I'm fit to have her back, and that would be it.

GETTING HELP

Most of the women I spoke to impressed me as being reluctant converts to probation. They had been initially suspicious, or even downright fearful, of being on probation. They had, however, come to see that there were benefits to be gained either by paying lip-service to the idea of probation or by accepting what they perceived to be a genuine offer of friendship and help from another individual who was 'nice' and who had access to certain resources (and who was coincidentally designated 'probation officer'). As Kevin Kirwin (1985:39) observes, 'being treated in a normal humane manner is often a pleasant surprise for...clients'.

Gwen was afraid that, in addition to the control exercised over her by her doctor, she would now be under surveillance by agents of the criminal justice system:

> I was very frightened of probation – I felt as though I was being owned by the police [sic]. I felt as though my life wasn't my own.

She had feared that being on probation would mean that she would have to forgo the right and the capacity to 'own' herself – that is, to define her own actions in the future. Such remarks also serve to explain why some women prefer to go to prison, despite the availability of apparently preferable alternatives.

But she, along with most of the others, appeared to have been won over by the 'helpfulness' of her particular probation officer. The process had started in court where, as Margaret Powell (1985:18) has stated, probation officers have traditionally been expected to 'offer immediate help – or at least a calm and clear explanation – to the distressed and uncomprehending' in court. Indeed, several of the women expressed appreciation of the presence of their probation officer in this bewildering setting:

> I could look at Mrs A and think there was a familiar face.

Later on in the relationship, 'helpfulness' was defined by the women in two ways: first, material help, and second, non-intrusive listening and advice-giving. In other words, the kind of help which the women looked for and appreciated most from their probation officers consisted of money (or at least help in obtaining it) and befriending.

Kirwin (1985:41) argues that probation officers frequently use their distrust of 'presenting problems' to justify refusing to undertake 'mundane' tasks for clients, such as 'phoning and writing to the DHSS, housing departments, and fuel boards or arranging nursery places'. Such 'mundane' tasks, however, may be daunting for women who are already lacking in confidence and self-esteem. A willingness by probation officers to use their professional authority and credibility (not to mention their telephones and postage) to negotiate with officialdom on their clients' behalf was certainly appreciated by the women, especially if there were no therapeutic 'strings' attached.

Apart from giving, or helping to obtain, material assistance, the most important function served by probation officers – according to the women – was that of alleviating loneliness. Being available, having time to listen – this was the service women wanted from their probation officers.

For two women, Maureen and Ivy, who already saw themselves as burdens on their own families, a sympathetic and disinterested listener was invaluable in preserving the remnants of family support:

> I can tell her anything...You can't tell your children – you've got to tell someone who's not involved. You don't want to foist your troubles on your family because they won't come and see me. They'll say, 'Oh, crikey – neurotic' – which perhaps I am.
>
> (Ivy)

> I like to come and talk to Mrs C. It's somebody to talk to and it's better than going blabbering and shouting your head off in the house.
>
> (Maureen)

It might be argued that, by befriending, probation officers are merely pandering to the ideology of the family, still allowing family members to channel all their problems on to 'mum', who then gets a probation officer to help her, instead of working with the whole family, 'helping them to understand the tremendous contradictory pressures placed upon them by the economic structures of capitalist society' (Corrigan and Leonard 1978: 29). In response, many probation officers would no doubt reply, 'It's all right for you to talk' (Cohen 1975) and continue with the one aspect of their role which appears to be rewarding for worker and client.

The building up of this relationship of trust, however, takes time. Pauline was experiencing her third probation order and described her probation officer thus:

> She's like an old friend and I know what she's like, so that now I trust her.

Eileen had known her probation officer even longer:

> I've been involved with Miss D since 1968...when I was 14. She's

been a great help – she's been involved fifteen years – we've got an understanding.

In the efficiency-conscious Probation Service of the 1980s, such a lengthy nurturance could hardly be justified as the most cost-effective use of officer resources. And there is, of course, no guarantee that such hard-won trust and understanding will actually prevent further criminal activity. As far as Pauline was concerned, the opposite seemed to be the case. Soon after I interviewed her, she committed a further offence.

A third way in which probation officers might be said to be of help to women was through *empowering*. Empowering consisted of providing the women with the kind of environment in which they could actually achieve something for themselves. *What* they achieved was not within the control of the probation officer – and sometimes it was not what the officer had originally intended. Nevertheless, the crucial characteristics of such provision was that it created a space in which the women were enabled to make some genuine choices, albeit within heavily circumscribed limits. In a small way, it allowed the women to exploit the gender contract in ways which were not self-defeating. Examples of this typically involved the creation of, or facilitating access to, work opportunities, though frequently such work was of a voluntary nature and the extent to which this served to keep the women in poverty must not be overlooked.

One logical extension of this empowering process was to allow women to do 'voluntary' work in order to discharge their obligations to the court. The issue of the appropriateness of Community Service for women is a vexed one (Dominelli 1984) but there was no doubt that the women I interviewed who had served such orders had not only thoroughly enjoyed their work, but had experienced a sense of achievement as well. Having admitted that she never paid fines, Carol said:

> The only thing I think they should give is Community Service, because you don't have to fork any money out and they don't have to fork money out (for prison). And I like working...I don't mind cleaning – I'll clean the whole house for you as long as you appreciate it.

On the other hand, one probation officer responsible for placing women in Community Service schemes felt that women fared better when they were not asked to do 'women's work', although he did feel that women might feel 'more comfortable' if such teams had women supervisors.

There is, therefore, a dilemma for the probation officer who wants to resist the prescriptive description of her/his female clients within the discourse of femininity. As can be seen from these accounts, many women are not seeking to break out of the ideologies that confine them to domesticity, sexual passivity, and sickness. Rather, they want to have the worst effects of those ideologies alleviated. The most appreciated probation officers were those who worked tactically to obtain material help, those who befriended in a one-to-one relationship, and those who provided part-time work opportunities which were role-appropriate (so that the women could feel confident in doing them well), relatively private and anonymous (so that the women did not feel conspicuous or stigmatized), and, above all, appreciated. Such findings appear to confirm those of Willis that 'Probation is primarily concerned with bringing relief and service to clients whose circumstances might have otherwise appeared to them intolerable...and this social work assistance is something clients both want and appreciate' (1986: 177). But individual solutions do not provide the alternative material and ideological conditions within which the women can constitute themselves differently – only collective political and policy solutions can do that.

CONCLUSION

From their own accounts, it is apparent that the women studied here experienced the criminal justice system as bewildering, degrading, and unjust. Yet their attempts to cope with it were characterized by neither total acceptance nor outright rejection of the treatment they received and the descriptions with which they were labelled. Rather, their attempts were characterized by accommodation – by a mixture of self-blame and suppressed anger, translated into a variety of petty resistances and rituals which might be conceived of as either 'shifting the signs' (Foucault 1975: 181) of the gender contract with a degree of agency or, alternatively, as 'minor deviations...[which] nurture the confined soul' (Ardener 1978: 29). These simple acts, it might be argued, because of the narrowness of the stage on which they are enacted, are of absorbing interest to the characters involved, but exert little influence on those who have the power to write the play.

But the attempts of these women to assert themselves and to take some control of their lives were steps which they had discovered for themselves and they were all the more precious for that. They represented their struggle to resist the constraints of both the ideological and the material conditions of their existence, which converged to confine them within domesticity, sexuality, and pathology. By doing contradictory things and exploiting the contradictions of the gender contract these women were rendering themselves 'nondescript' and could be seen as having taken the first steps towards breaking out of such confines.

Chapter Nine

WOMEN OFFENDERS OR OFFENDING WOMEN?

This book is a case study in social control and its resistance. Its aim has been two-fold:

– to analyse the production of a certain group of female law-breakers as 'nondescript women'; that is, women who, because they do not 'fit' any professionally defined categories, are largely both neglected by, and to some extent free of, professional control;

– to describe the ideological and material conditions which underpin this production and which allow this group of offending women to stand in a metonymical relationship to certain other women who, while they may not break the law, nevertheless offend against – and are offended by – the accepted norms of femininity.

WOMEN OFFENDERS

The thesis of this study is that certain women are muted within the criminal justice system. They are subject to multiple discursive oppression which is subtle and sophisticated. Their oppression is dependent not on their active and constant domination by one group (men) in society but by the inability and/or refusal of a number of authorized definers (who, empirically, may be either men or women) to hear or listen to communications which are incongruent with professionally legitimated modes of expression about female conditions of existence. Consequently, the women are disqualified as speakers about their own condition and are, instead, strategically constructed as the programmable objects of professional discourses. They are effectively offered a contract which promises to minimize the consequences of their criminality by rehabilitating them within the dominant discourses of femininity (that is, domesticity, sexuality, and pathology). Despite these programmes of feminization, such women, it is argued, attempt to resist such construction by exploiting the contradictions of official discourses. As a result, the 'experts' find such women impossible to define and they appear to be beyond definition both as women and as criminals. Yet, while much of the women's resistance is individualistic, inconsistent, and, in some senses, self-destructive, it has the important effect of undermining the authority of official discourses and keeping open the possibility of the creation of new knowledge about them – both as women and as law-breakers.

In order to understand the 'subtle and sophisticated' ways in which some women experience oppression in the criminal justice process, this study has offered a critique of the various discourses which lay claim to knowledge about female law-breakers. Statements made by those medical, judicial, and welfare personnel whose job it is to assess, judge, defend, treat, and punish nondescript women have been deconstructed. It has been argued that:

1) Magistrates' discourse in general is constituted by the ideology of common sense and the material conditions of a privileged existence. Additionally, women magistrates are required simultaneously to claim (for the purposes of authoritative understanding) and deny (for the purposes of authoritative attribution of culpability) similarity with female law-breakers.

2) Solicitors' discourse is constituted by the ideology of legal representation which requires solicitors to repackage female law-breakers according to typifications of 'normal' women which can be discursively recognized by 'magisterial common sense'.

3) Psychiatrists' discourse is constituted by the ideology of forensic medicine, which requires and authorizes psychiatrists to make wide-ranging medical, moral, and judicial judgements of female law-breakers in order to render them describable for the purposes of recognition by 'magisterial common sense'. At the same time, this ideology makes women's eligibility for treatment both ideologically and materially dependent on a far narrower range of gender-stereotyped classifications.

4) Probation officers' discourse is constituted, on the one hand, by the competing discourses of magistrates, solicitors, and psychiatrists who, having failed to describe these women adequately within their own discourses, often reach consensus about the competence of probation officers to describe them. On the other hand (and simultaneously), probation officers' discourse is constituted within a social work ideology, which requires and authorizes them both to care for and to control women as key figures in the maintenance of the nuclear family (whether or not the women are, in fact, members of such families).

The fundamental object of this study, however, has been neither to apportion blame to 'experts' for their 'failures' to encapsulate law-breaking women in expert discourses nor to 'celebrate' the women's resistances as being essentially liberative. Rather, it has been to suggest how both 'experts' and female law-breakers are struggling to make sense of the contradictions between formal criminal justice in particular and substantive social justice in general.

But critique has its limitations (Rose 1987) and, as Cohen (1983: 126) argues, while we should not be deceived by appearance, neither should we perhaps be obsessed with debunking. Is it possible, or indeed desirable, to 'read off' from critique solutions to the problems identified? Or is the writer forever confined to saying to those of whom she writes, 'I have discovered the contradictions in what you say, I have unearthed the rules and structures which explain why you say it, I have demonstrated its consequences for others, but ultimately you have no alternative because the discourses available to you allow you to speak and act no differently'?

Such pessimism about the possibility of change is not, however, wholly justified. To demonstrate the inextricable link between power and knowledge is not to imply that the only relationship that can exist between 'experts' and those they define is one of domination and submission. The recognition that 'the power of expertise installs a new type of relation between authority and its subjects' (Rose 1987: 74), coupled with an understanding of power relations as local and immanent, allows for the possibility of a redistribution of power – albeit in an uneven and paradoxical fashion. Precisely because of the variety and competitiveness of expert discourses, it is possible to exploit contradictions and work tactically in ways which need not oppress. Because, as Rose asserts, 'pluralism is more than a myth' (1987: 73), it is possible for women offenders to be empowered by experts, although the ways in which this can be done do not sit easily under ideologically 'sound' banners. For, as Cohen (1983) argues, one ideology can be used to support quite different policies and one policy can be supported for very different ideological reasons. There are no easy answers, but there are some difficult and compromising value decisions to be made by professionals at both an individual and policy level.

OFFENDING WOMEN?

As Carlen (1988: 3) has pointed out, 'women...are on the whole a law-abiding lot'. But, while the production and reproduction of 'nondescriptiveness' among female law-breakers is made possible by a particular constellation of material and ideological conditions, the experiences of these particular women offer insights into the experience of all women. Techniques of muting can be recognized as much by the law-abiding woman as by the law-breaker. The dissemination of authorized versions of what constitutes reality, the blunting of self-perceptions through the encouragement of 'trivial' concerns and small-scale pleasures, and tacit exclusion from 'public' space comprise the routine frustrations of many women's lives. Expert scripts are to be found acted out as frequently in the doctor's surgery, the headteacher's study, the hairdresser's salon, and the car mechanic's garage as in the court-room, as many women will testify.

What, then, are the routine components of such muting scripts which serve to render women invisible, guilty, treatable, and manageable? Anne Dickson (1982) neatly describes the situation in which so many women find themselves as the 'compassion trap'. 'The compassion trap is usually defined as a sense of obligation that, as a woman, you should put everyone else's needs before your own all of the time. You should always be available and accessible to others' (Dickson 1982: 54). She continues to provide numerous examples of ways in which women fall into the compassion trap in their day-to-day interactions with strangers and friends, both at home and at work:

165

the patient who doesn't want to worry the overworked nurses with a request for medication...the woman who reluctantly accepts a new hairstyle because she doesn't want to offend the enthusiastic new stylist...the woman who has sex with her boyfriend because he is turned on and she feels sorry for him... the woman who has sacrificed her whole career to look after her invalid parents...the secretary who will not tell her boss he has made a mistake because it might deflate his ego.

(Dickson 1982: 55-6)

And so on and so on. Dickson argues that women tend to respond to such demands in ways which are understandable but ultimately destructive, both of themselves and of others. They tend to lurch between passivity and aggressiveness, the latter being expressed in two ways – either directly, or indirectly in the form of manipulative emotional blackmail. By contrast, Dickson advocates 'assertiveness as a way of life' (1982: 154). Assertiveness is achieving congruence between what you feel and what you communicate. It involves:

a) accepting, recognizing, and understanding what you feel;
b) learning to express what you feel clearly and confidently without manipulating or oppressing others; and
c) accepting responsibility for your feelings, what you say, and the consequences of both.

Helpful as Dickson's book undoubtedly is, it makes a basic assumption which is untenable within any structural analysis of women's experiences. 'Being assertively powerful,' she argues, 'starts with being yourself' (1982: 147). This book, by contrast, has argued that 'being yourself' is a luxury which is unavailable to the women in this study and to many women in our society. Indeed, the representation of the subject in various discourses and before various institutions as a social agent having a unitary form has been rejected. Instead, subjects have been viewed as 'the differentiated terminals of the varied capacities and practices they engage in' (Hirst and Woolley 1982: 120).

The implication of such an analysis is that resistance to social control takes many forms, none of which is inherently better than any other, and all of which merit recognition and analysis within the socio-economic context through which they emerge. The

166

ultimate irony, it seems, would be for women to feel guilty about not being assertive. Scripts which render women invisible, unnoticed, and lacking authority or credibility also, in some contexts, allow them to go unnoticed, to elude authority, and to get away with incredible actions. Scripts which blame women or encourage them to feel guilty, inadequate, or unworthy can also, in some contexts, allow them to make demands on those who profess to offer help to the 'inadequate'. Likewise, being viewed as 'sick' and in need of treatment is a script which can be turned to one's advantage in avoiding arduous responsibilities. And, finally, scripts which render women manageable by circumscribing their activities, channelling their energies into trivial pursuits, and encouraging satisfaction in small-scale pleasures may also allow some women to act out some part of their lives with frustrating autonomy since, ironically, official discourse frequently has power only to draw the boundaries and not to prescribe the content of such activities.

One of the aims of this book has been to challenge the traditional boundaries between women who break the law and women who do not. In so doing it has tried to avoid, on the one hand, trite arguments about 'hidden' criminality and, on the other, assertions about the universal oppression of women – assertions which may or may not be true, but which are unhelpful in understanding the significant minutiae of the differences which constitute women's experiences. Instead, it has attempted to demonstrate the variety of ways in which women are subject to social control through the claims of expertise or professional knowledge and to give credence to the equal variety of ways (many of which may not be regarded as appropriately assertive or 'ideologically sound') in which women seek to – and often succeed in – resisting such control.

APPENDIX:
RESEARCHING WOMEN

For this study, I gathered a number of statements from the following sources:

1) Interviews with the following sixty-four people who had experience of working with women law-breakers:

– twenty-nine probation officers (working in probation offices, hostels, and prison)
– eight solicitors
– twelve magistrates
– seven psychiatrists
– eight 'miscellaneous' individuals, e.g. a psychiatric community nurse, an ex-prison officer, a couple of court clerks.

2) Interviews with eleven female law-breakers subject to probation investigation, probation orders, or community service orders, nine of whom had also experienced psychiatric assessment or treatment.

3) Notes from the case records of these, and other, female law-breakers, made available to me by probation officers. I approached approximately 100 people; the ways in which I approached them and their responses are explained below.

PROBATION OFFICERS

I was given permission by the Chief Probation Officer of Staffordshire to approach any staff within two Assistant Chief Probation Officer areas (there were four in all in Staffordshire) – one entirely urban and one a mixture of the urban and rural. I examined the most recent statistical returns for these two areas and identified those probation officers who carried *either* any cases of women subject to probation orders with psychiatric conditions *or* four or more women subject to supervision of any kind of criminal offences. I supposed (not always correctly) that officers in the latter category might have a particular interest in working with women law-breakers, since there is at least some element of choice exercised by officers in selecting their own cases. A total of thirty-seven officers fell into those categories (out of sixty-two in those areas) Letters were sent to all thirty-seven and twenty-eight agreed to be interviewed. One additional officer sent written comments in reply to my letter. Of the twenty-eight interviewed, three did not wish to be recorded on tape but the remaining twenty-five agreed to this also. (The transcripts of most recorded interviews are available as part of my PhD thesis (Worrall 1987b).)

I also contacted probation officers working in five hostels catering for women and two women's prisons in the region. I received positive responses from three hostels and four officers working in prisons. Interviews with probation officers varied in length from thirty to ninety minutes.

MAGISTRATES

Access to magistrates was obtained through a magistrates' clerk with whom I had worked in the past. He identified for me a total of eighteen magistrates who were members of a local probation committee and had attended a meeting which I had addressed on the subject of 'Female Offenders'. Letters were sent to all eighteen. Of these, four sent written comments in reply and eight agreed to be interviewed. None of these interviews was tape-recorded. Two of them took place in workplaces, where taping would not have been possible. The rest were conducted in homes, where 'serious' discussion was interspersed with 'chit-chat', coffee, lunch, and visitors; a request to tape would have seemed discourteous, I felt.

SOLICITORS

I wrote to nine solicitors known to me as a probation officer. Of these, two sent written comments in reply and six agreed to be interviewed. Only one interview (with the only female solicitor) was taped. One of the other interviews was conducted over lunch, while the other interviewees impressed me as either too intimidating or too intimidated to be asked.

PSYCHIATRISTS

I wrote to a total of eight consultant psychiatrists, some known to me from previous contact in the Probation Service and some recommended to me by other interviewees. I had not expected a positive response from this group and was therefore pleasantly surprised when one sent written comments and six agreed to be interviewed. Of these, two specialized in forensic psychiatry and the remaining five were general psychiatrists. Of the six interviews, three were tape-recorded, one declined to be taped, and the remaining two were not asked, because I was clearly being 'fitted into' a busy day and interruptions were likely to be frequent.

MISCELLANEOUS INTERVIEWS AND CONTACTS

A small number of other interviews were conducted and contacts attempted. A psychiatric community nurse working with an interviewed probation officer agreed to give a tape-recorded interview. Two psychiatric nurses working in a women's prison agreed to be interviewed during my visit. Three magistrates' clerks agreed to be interviewed (two of them in a joint interview). A letter placed in a local newspaper produced a response from an ex-prison officer (female) as well as an ex-offender. A letter placed in *Probation Journal* produced replies from three interested serving probation officers but, unfortunately, follow-up questionnaires were not returned. Finally, I interviewed the organizer of a voluntary counselling service for women charged with shoplifting.

FEMALE LAW-BREAKERS

The only realistic way of gaining access to this group was through their probation officers (a letter in a local newspaper elicited only one response). At the end of each interview with a probation officer, I discussed the possibility of interviewing one or more of the women they had discussed. I had prepared a letter which I asked the officer to give to the woman concerned, explaining the purpose of my research and inviting her to be interviewed. She could return the letter either directly to me or via her probation officer. I offered to see her at home or at a probation office and assured her that her probation officer could be present, or not, as she wished. If s/he were not present they would not be told about the details of the interview.

During interviews, it became clear that a number of officers did not want me to interview their clients. Reasons commonly given were about practicalities ('It's difficult to pin her down'), recent crises ('She's in a real mess at the moment and won't want the pressure'), ignorance ('She wouldn't understand who you are or what you're doing'), and relationships ('She's very suspicious'). It was perhaps understandable that 'recommended' clients were those with whom the officer felt s/he had established at least an element of rapport and trust. It takes more than a little courage to expose to 'scientific' gaze those relationships where mistrust, hostility, and disappointment seem to be the overwhelming characteristics. I was also sensitive to the fear (tactfully unexpressed) that *I* might ruin carefully worked-at relationships.

In the event, fifteen women were identified as 'appropriate' but only ten were eventually interviewed (plus the one who responded to the newspaper letter). Of the remaining five, two failed to keep appointments (one on two occasions). In the other three cases, the officers, after initially agreeing to approach the women, later felt they could not do so because of 'new crises'. Of the eleven interviews finally conducted, eight were tape-recorded. One of the remaining interviews was conducted in a café, one on a hospital ward, and one in the unavoidable presence of other people who were not fully aware of the purpose of my visit but would have become very suspicious if I had produced my tape recorder.

In total, then, I conducted seventy-five interviews, ranging in length from fifteen minutes to two and a half hours. Of those, forty-one were tape-recorded, and thirty-four later transcribed. Notes were made at the time of, or very soon after, the remaining thirty. In addition, eight people sent written comments in reply to my letters. Twenty-four people either declined to be interviewed or failed to respond to my request.

LETTER TO WOMEN

Dear

I am writing to ask if you would help me with some research I am doing at Keele University. I am talking to women who are on Probation, or Community Service Orders, to see what they expected to happen when they went to court and what they think about what has happened to them since then. Mr X has given me permission to write to you but if you do not want to take part in this research, that is entirely up to you – it will not affect your Community Service reports. However, if you do agree to see me, I understand that the time you spend will be counted towards your Order.

If you are prepared to help me, please complete the slip below and give it to Mr X. I will meet you at your nearest Probation Office or at your home and there will not be anyone else present, unless you wish. Anything you tell me will be treated confidentially.

Thank you very much for reading this letter.

Yours sincerely,

Anne Worrall

....

I am willing to help with your research.

You may see me at .... Probation Office, or at my home (cross out whichever does not apply)

The most convenient times to see me are:

Signed ....

Address...

172

LETTER TO MAGISTRATES

Dear

The Deputy Clerk to the Justices, Mr A, has kindly given me your name, as I understand that you attended a talk I gave in September last year on 'Female Offenders'. I believe I mentioned then that I am continuing my research into this subject as a postgraduate student at Keele. I have been interviewing a number of Probation Officers, solicitors and women offenders, but would be most grateful to hear the views of magistrates who have some experience of dealing with women.

I am wondering, therefore, whether you would be prepared to spare me a little time (15–30 minutes would suffice) to discuss any, or all, of the following questions:

1. In your experience, are there particular problems associated with trying and sentencing women?

2. In your experience, would you expect Social Enquiry Reports and Psychiatric Reports to play a greater or lesser part in sentencing women than men?

3. In your experience, do courts treat women more or less sympathetically than men, or does it vary – in which case – how?

I am available to come and see you most days between 9.30 a.m. and 3.30 p.m., but I appreciate that this may not be the most convenient time of day for you. If it is more convenient, I would be happy to 'catch' you in a free moment at the Magistrates' Court, or, alternatively, I would be grateful for any written comments on the above points. Obviously, any views you feel able to express would be treated confidentially.

I enclose a stamped addressed envelope for your reply. Thank you for considering my request.

Yours sincerely,

Anne Worrall

LETTER TO SOLICITORS

Dear

I am a former Probation Officer, currently undertaking postgraduate research at Keele University into 'Community Provision for Female Offenders'. I have interviewed a number of Probation Officers and women clients, but would be most grateful to hear the views of some members of the legal profession and the judiciary who have experience of dealing with women.

I am wondering, therefore, whether you would be prepared to spare me a little time (15 – 20 minutes would suffice) to discuss any, or all, of the following questions:

1. In your experience, are there particular problems associated with prosecuting, defending, or sentencing women?

2. In your experience, would you expect Social Enquiry Reports and/or Psychiatric Reports to be prepared on women more or less frequently than on men?

3. In your experience, do Courts treat women more or less sympathetically than men, or does it vary – in which case – how?

If you feel unable to see me, I would be most grateful for any written comments. Obviously, any views you feel able to express will be treated confidentially.

Thank you for considering my request.

Yours sincerely,

Anne Worrall

LETTER TO PSYCHIATRISTS

Dear

I am a former Probation Officer, currently undertaking postgraduate research at Keele University into 'Community Provision for Mentally Disordered Female Offenders'. I have interviewed a number of Probation Officers and women clients, but would be most grateful to hear the views of psychiatrists who have experience of preparing reports on female offenders for courts and undertaking treatment of women subject to court orders.

I am wondering, therefore, whether you or any of your colleagues would be prepared to spare me a little time (15–30 minutes would suffice) to discuss any, or all, of the following questions:

1. In your experience, are most of the women on whom you are asked to prepare court reports suffering from treatable mental disorders?

2. In your experience, are court orders for psychiatric treatment (in-patient or out-patient) ever made against your recommendation or without consulting you? Is there any difference between men and women in this respect?

3. In your experience, are there particular problems associated with treating people subject to court orders? Is there any difference between men and women in this respect?

I appreciate that your time is valuable and I would be prepared to see you at any time between 9.30 am and 3.30 pm. If you feel unable to see me, I would be most grateful for any written comments. Obviously any views you feel able to express will be treated confidentially.

I enclose a stamped addressed envelope for your reply. Thank you for considering this request.

Yours sincerely,

Anne Worrall

LETTER TO PROBATION OFFICERS

Dear

You may be aware that I am currently undertaking research at Keele University into community provision for adult female offenders. I see from recent County statistics that you have a number of women on your caseload and I am wondering whether you would be prepared to allow me to interview you about them. I am particularly interested in any women who have, at any time, been diagnosed as mentally disordered (especially ....) but I would also like to ask you some general questions about your work with women. If you can spare me some time (about 30 minutes), perhaps you would be kind enough to return the slip below, giving two or three alternative times that are convenient to you between now and..... If you feel unable to spare this time, I would be most grateful if you would be prepared to complete the attached questionnaire.

If you have any further questions, I can be contacted on the above telephone number (Mondays are best) or on ... in the evenings.

Thank you very much for your co-operation.

Yours sincerely,

Anne Worrall

....

I shall be available for interview

on	1.	at	am/pm
or	2.	at	am/pm
or	3.	at	am/pm

I do/do not object to this interview being tape-recorded (strictly for the purpose of research).

Signed ....
Address....................................
....
....

INTERVIEW SCHEDULE FOR PROBATION OFFICERS

1. I am interested in finding out how Probation Officers feel about their women clients – do you have many on your caseload?

2. How did they come to be under supervision?

3. What have you been doing to try and help them?

4. Have you had to contact other agencies for them? (Doctors, DHSS etc.)

5. What have been these other agencies' attitudes towards them?

6. Have you wanted to obtain specific services for them? (Jobs, money, housing, nursery places etc.)

7. Have you had any problems in obtaining these services?

8. Do you think that this is the right agency to deal with the women you have mentioned?

9. Do you think that women clients, in general, present any special problems for Probation Officers?

10. Have you had any woman on your caseload who has given you particular problems? Could you tell me about her?

NOTES

INTRODUCTION

1. The term *nondescript* is used throughout this book to refer to the product of the processes which subject particular female law-breakers to inappropriate and unsuccessful judicial and welfare needs to categorize them within the discourses of femininity – processes in which the women themselves play an active, if limited, part.

CHAPTER TWO

1. This study is concerned primarily with the treatment of women in magistrates' courts, although several of the women discussed (notably Kathy) had been dealt with at the Crown Court at some time.
2. The most significant powers of the courts in relation to mentally disordered offenders are as follow:
a) *Diminished Responsibility* (Homicide Act 1957, s.2), which has the effect of reducing a charge of murder to one of manslaughter, thus increasing the court's sentencing discretion.
b) *Provisions under the Mental Health Act 1983*, most notably:
   – s. 35, which permits a *remand* to hospital (instead of prison) for the purposes of preparing medical and social inquiry reports;
   – s. 37, which *sentences* an offender to a Hospital Order (initially for six months, with the possibility of renewal);
   – s. 41, which *sentences* an offender to a Hospital Order for a fixed or unlimited period, but from which discharge is restricted by the consent of the Home Secretary or a Mental Health Review Tribunal;
   – s. 47, which permits a prisoner to be transferred *post-sentence* from prison to hospital.
c) *Probation Order* with a condition of in-patient or out-patient treatment (Powers of the Courts Act 1973, s.3) for a fixed time or for the duration of the probation order, with the consent of the defendant.

Of these provisions, only sections 35 and 37 of the Mental Health Act 1983 and a probation order with condition of treatment are available to magistrates' courts.

3. Magistrates' courts have the power to adjourn a case after conviction and before sentence for up to four weeks for the purpose of enabling enquiries to be made or for determining the most suitable method of dealing with the case (Criminal Justice Act 1967, s. 30). Reports are prepared on a more routine basis for the Crown Courts and a Home Office Circular in 1971 (59/1971) identified *any* woman defendant as a particular category on which reports should be prepared. That circular was only overridden in 1986 by Circular 92/1986. Many probation officers would now acknowledge that the routine emphasis on the role expectations of 'normal' womanhood in social inquiry reports on female offenders disadvantages many women who do not readily fit those stereotypes. It has also been suggested recently (Mair and Brockington 1988) that, since the very existence of a report may push a defendant 'up tariff' and since women are more likely to be referred for a report than men, the preparation of reports may, of itself, indirectly discriminate against women.

CHAPTER THREE

1. For more detailed discussion of the 'Gender Contract', see 'Introduction' by Pat Carlen and Anne Worrall in Carlen and Worrall (1987).

2. At the time of these interviews in 1983, I was not myself as acutely conscious of racism as an issue to be considered in the treatment of offenders as I have since become and did not, therefore, raise it in any of my discussions. I now see this as an obvious weakness in the study.

CHAPTER FOUR

1. Most magistrates made an almost automatic link between fines and television licence offences and several expressed concern that women were discriminated against in respect of this particular offence, since they were often the ones at home during the day when detector officials called. Television was seen by magistrates as 'part of the family' and women tended to receive sympathy for what amounted to an additional domestic responsibility. See note to Chapter Five for further discussion of this point.

2. At the time of this research, detention centres existed for young men but not young women. Since the Criminal Justice Act 1988, there is virtually no formal difference in provision for men and women offenders. However, in practice, there are very few attendance centres or Intermediate Treatment schemes for young women and

those serving sentences in young offender institutions frequently mix with older women prisoners – a practice discouraged in relation to young men.

3. This relationship has been largely neglected by the literature about magistrates' courts, although two articles have intimated that it may have some special significance (Farrington and Morris 1983; Dominelli 1984). In both articles it is suggested that women magistrates may be less lenient than their male colleagues in their sentencing of women and that this punitive disposition may be attributable to a sense of affront. Women who break the law, it is argued, are censured by women magistrates for their 'betrayal' of womanhood. I have attempted to demonstrate that the process whereby women in court – both magistrates and defendants – are muted is rather more complex than that (see also Worrall 1987b).

CHAPTER FIVE

1. Sensitivity to gynaecological mitigations appears to be selective. Menopause and pregnancy may mitigate a shoplifting offence but not, apparently, a motoring offence, where women are regarded as asexual. Motoring is evidently a world which women must enter on men's terms or not at all. There may be a number of reasons for this. Magistrates' sentencing discretion is more restricted in this area and it is normal practice to standardize sentences in a particular court on a particular day, regardless of the characteristics of individual defendants. The same, incidentally, applies to television licence offences but the inequity of this practice seems to be more readily acknowledged. For further discussion of this point see Worrall 1987a.

CHAPTER SIX

1. The Special Treatment Unit is the anonymized name of a unit attached to a local psychiatric hospital and specializing in the treatment of people diagnosed as suffering from 'personality disorders'.

CHAPTER SEVEN

1. For further discussion of the policy and practice implications of this analysis for probation officers see my article in the *British Journal of Social Work* (Worrall 1989).

BIBLIOGRAPHY

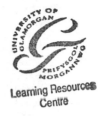

Learning Resources
Centre

Adler, Z. (1987) *Rape on Trial*, London: Routledge & Kegan Paul.

Allen, H. (1986) 'Psychiatry and the construction of the feminine' in P. Miller and N. Rose (eds) *The Power of Psychiatry*, Cambridge: Polity Press.

Allen, H. (1987a) 'Rendering them harmless: the professional portrayal of women charged with serious violent crimes' in P. Carlen and A. Worrall (eds) *Gender, Crime and Justice*, Milton Keynes: Open University Press.

Allen, H. (1987b) *Justice Unbalanced*, Milton Keynes: Open University Press.

Ardener, S. (1978) *Defining Women*, London: Croom Helm.

Ashworth, A. and Gostin, L. (1984) 'Mentally disordered offenders and the sentencing process', *The Criminal Law Review* 195–212.

Bailey, R. and Brake, M. (eds) (1975) *Radical Social Work*, London: Arnold.

Baldwin, J. and Bottomley, A.K. (eds) (1978) *Criminal Justice*, London: Martin Robertson.

Baldwin, J. and McConville, M. (1977) *Negotiated Justice*, London: Martin Robertson.

Bankowski, Z.K., Hutton, N.R., and McManus, J.J. (1987) *Lay Justice?* Edinburgh: T. & T. Clark.

Barker, P. (1986) *Basic Family Therapy*, London: Collins.

Barrett, M. and McIntosh, M. (1982) *The Anti-Social Family*, London: Verso.

Blythe, R. (1969) *Akenfield*, London: Allen Lane.

Bottoms, A. and McClean, J. (1976) *Defendants in the Criminal Process*, London: Routledge & Kegan Paul.

Bottoms, A and McWilliams, W. (1979) 'A non-treatment paradigm for probation practice', *British Journal of Social Work* 9 (2): 159–202.

Box, S. (1983) *Power, Crime and Mystification*, London: Tavistock.

Brook, E. and Davis, A. (eds) (1985) *Women, The Family and Social Work*, London: Tavistock.

Brophy, J. and Smart, C. (eds) (1985) *Women in Law*, London: Routledge & Kegan Paul.

Burney, E. (1979) *J.P: Magistrate, Court and Community*, London: Hutchinson.

Burton, F. and Carlen, P. (1979) *Official Discourse*, London: Routledge & Kegan Paul.

Calvert, J. (1985) 'Motherhood', in E. Brook and A. Davis (eds) *Women, The Family and Social Work*, London: Tavistock.

Carlen, P. (1976) *Magistrates' Justice*, Oxford: Martin Robertson.

Carlen, P. (1983) *Women's Imprisonment*, London: Routledge & Kegan Paul.

Carlen, P. (1985) 'Introduction', in P. Carlen *et al. Criminal Women*, Cambridge: Polity Press.

Carlen, P. (1986) 'Psychiatry in prisons: promises, premises, practices and politics', in P. Miller and N. Rose (eds) *The Power of Psychiatry*, Cambridge: Polity Press.

Carlen, P. (1988) *Women, Crime and Poverty*, Milton Keynes: Open University Press.

Carlen, P. and Collison, M. (eds) (1980) *Radical Issues in Criminology*, Oxford: Martin Robertson.

Carlen, P., Hicks, J., O'Dwyer, J., Christina, D., and Tchaikowsky, C. (1985) *Criminal Women*, Cambridge: Polity Press.

Carlen, P. and Worrall, A. (eds) (1987) *Gender, Crime and Justice*, Milton Keynes: Open University Press.

Chesler, P. (1974) *Women and Madness*, London: Allen Lane.

Cicourel, A.V. (1968) *The Social Organisation of Juvenile Justice*, New York: Wiley.

Cohen, S. (1975) 'It's all right for you to talk: political and sociological manifesto for social work action', in R. Bailey and M. Brake (eds) *Radical Social Work*, London: Arnold.

Cohen, S. (1983) 'Social control talk: telling stories about correctional change', in D. Garland and P. Young (eds) *The Power to Punish*, London: Heinemann.

Cook, D. (1987) 'Women on welfare: in crime or injustice?, in P. Carlen and A. Worrall (eds) *Gender, Crime and Justice*, Milton Keynes: Open University Press.

Corrigan, P. and Leonard, P. (1978) *Social Work Practice Under Capitalism: A Marxist Approach*, London: Macmillan.

Cousins, M. (1978) 'The logic of deconstruction', *Oxford Literary Review* 3 (2): 70–7.

Cousins, M. and Hussain, A. (1984) *Michel Foucault*, London: Macmillan.

Culler, J. (1976) *Saussure*, London: Fontana.

Dell, S. (1971) *Silent in Court*, London: Bell.

Dickson, A. (1982) *A Woman in Your Own Right*, London: Quartet Books.

Dobash, R. and Dobash, R.E. (1979) *Violence Against Wives*, London: Open Books.

Dominelli, L. (1984) 'Differential justice: domestic labour, community service and female offenders', *Probation Journal* 31 (3): 100–3.

Donzelot, J. (1979) *The Policing of Families*, London: Hutchinson.

Downes, D.M. and Rock, P. (eds) (1979) *Deviant Interpretations*, Oxford:

Downes, D.M. and Rock, P. (eds) (1979) *Deviant Interpretations*, Oxford: Martin Robertson.

Eaton, M. (1985) 'Documenting the defendant: placing women in social inquiry reports', in J. Brophy and C. Smart (eds) *Women in Law*, London: Routledge & Kegan Paul.

Eaton, M. (1987) 'The question of bail: magistrates' responses to applications for bail on behalf of men and women defendants', in P. Carlen and A. Worrall (eds) *Gender, Crime and Justice*, Milton Keynes: Open University Press.

Edwards, S. (1981) *Female Sexuality and the Law*, Oxford: Martin Robertson.

Edwards, S. (1984) *Women on Trial*, Manchester: Manchester University Press.

Edwards, S. (ed.) (1985) *Gender, Sex and the Law*, London: Croom Helm.

Ehrenreich, B. and English, D. (1973) *Complaints and Disorders*, London: Writers & Readers.

Eichenbaum, L. and Orbach, S. (1982) *Outside In, Inside Out*, Harmondsworth: Pelican.

Family Policy Studies Centre (1984) *One-Parent Families*, Fact Sheet, London: Family Policy Studies Centre.

Farrington, D. and Morris, A. (1983) 'Sex, sentencing and reconviction', *British Journal of Criminology* 23 (3): 123–35.

Foucault, M. (1965) *Madness and Civilization*, London: Tavistock.

Foucault, M. (1972) *The Archaeology of Knowledge*, London: Tavistock.

Foucault, M. (1973) *The Birth of the Clinic*, London: Tavistock.

Foucault, M. (1975) *I, Pierre Rivière....*, New York: Pantheon.

Garfinkel, H. (1968) *Studies in Ethnomethodology*, Englewood Cliffs, NJ: Prentice-Hall.

Garland, D. (1985) *Punishment and Welfare*, Aldershot: Gower.

Garland, D. and Young, P. (eds) (1983) *The Power to Punish*, London: Heinemann.

Gibbens, T., Soothill, K., and Pope, P. (1977) *Medical Remands in Criminal Courts*, Oxford: Oxford University Press.

Glover, E. (1969) *The Psychopathology of Prostitution*, London: Institute for the Study and Treatment of Delinquency.

Gordon, C. (1977) 'Birth of the subject', *Radical Philosophy* 17: 15–25.

Gordon, C. (1979) 'Other inquisitions', *Ideology and Consciousness* 6: 23–46.

Harris, R. (1980) 'A changing service: the case for separating care and control in probation practice', *British Journal of Social Work* 10 (2): 163–84.

Hay, D. (1975) 'Property, authority and the criminal law', in D. Hay *et al.* (eds) *Albion's Fatal Tree*, London: Allen Lane.

Hay, D., Linebaugh, P., and Thompson, E.P. (eds) (1975) *Albion's Fatal Tree*, London: Allen Lane.

Heberling, J.L. (1978) 'Plea negotiation in England', in J. Baldwin and A.K. Bottomley (eds) *Criminal Justice*, London: Martin Robertson.

Heidensohn, F. (1985) *Women and Crime*, London: Macmillan.

Hewitt, M. (1983) 'Bio-politics and social policy: Foucault's account of welfare', *Theory, Culture and Society* 2 (1): 67–84.

Hindelang, M.J. (1979) 'Sex differences in criminal activity', *Social Problems* 27: 143–56.

Hirst, P. (1980) 'Law, socialism and rights', in P. Carlen and M. Collison (eds) *Radical Issues in Criminology*, Oxford: Martin Robertson.

Hirst, P. and Woolley, P. (1982) *Social Relations and Human Attributes*, London: Tavistock.

Home Office (1983) *Report of the Work of the Prison Department*, Cmnd. 9306, London: HMSO.

Home Office (1984) *Probation Service in England and Wales: Statement of National Objectives and Priorities*, London: Home Office.

Home Office (1986a) *The Sentence of the Court*, London: HMSO.

Home Office (1986b) *Probation Statistics, England and Wales, 1984*, London: HMSO.

Hood, R. (1962) *Sentencing in Magistrates' Courts*, London: Stevens.

Hudson, B. (1984) 'Femininity and adolescence', in A. McRobbie and M. Nava (eds) *Gender and Generation*, Basingstoke: Macmillan.

Huntington, J. (1981) *Social Work and General Medical Practice: Collaboration or Conflict?*, London: Allen Unwin.

Hutter, B. and Williams, G. (eds) (1981) *Controlling Women*, London: Croom Helm.

Kirwin, K. (1985) 'Probation and supervision', in H. Walker and B. Beaumont (eds) *Working with Offenders*, London: Macmillan.

Klein, D. and Kress, D. (1976) 'Any woman's blues', *Crime and Social Justice*, spring–summer: 34–49.

Kristeva, J. (1975) 'The system and the speaking subject', in T.A. Sebeok (ed.) *The Tell-Tale Sign*, Peter de Ridder Press.

Lees, S. (1986) 'Sex, race and culture: feminism and the limits of cultural pluralism', *Feminist Review* 22: 92–101.

Lewis, P. (1980) *Psychiatric Probation Orders*, Cambridge: University of Cambridge Institute of Criminology.

Lombroso, C. and Ferrero, W. (1959) *The Female Offender*, New York: Peter Owen Ltd., originally published in 1895.

London Borough of Brent (1985) *A Child in Trust*, London: London Borough of Brent.

Luckhaus, L. (1985) 'A plea for PMT in the criminal law', in S. Edwards (ed.) *Gender, Sex and the Law*, London: Croom Helm.

McBarnet, D. (1981) 'Magistrates' courts and the ideology of justice', *British Journal of Law and Society* 8 (2): 181–97.

McGuire, M. and Priestley, P. (1985) *Offending Behaviour*, London: Batsford.

McLeod, E. (1982) *Women Working: Prostitution Now*, London: Croom Helm.

McRobbie, A. and Nava, M. (eds) (1984) *Gender and Generation*, Basingstoke: Macmillan.

Mair, G. and Brockington, N. (1988) 'Female offenders and the probation service', *The Howard Journal of Criminal Justice* 27 (2): 117–26.

Mathiesen, T. (1972) *The Defences of the Weak*, London: Tavistock, first published in 1965.

Mead, G.H. (1934) *On Social Psychology*, Chicago: University of Chicago Press.

Messerschmidt, J. (1987) *Capitalism, Patriarchy and Crime: Towards a Socialist Feminist Criminology*, Totowa, NJ: Rowan & Littlefield.

Millard, D.A. (1982) 'Keeping the probation service whole: the case for discretion', *British Journal of Social Work* 12: 291–301.

Miller, J.B. (1976) *Towards a New Psychology of Women*, Harmondsworth: Pelican.

Miller, P. and Rose, N. (eds) (1986) *The Power of Psychiatry*, Cambridge: Polity Press.

Mitchell, J.C. (1983) 'Case and situation analysis', *Sociological Review* 33: 187–211.

National Association for the Care and Resettlement of Offenders (1983) *Women in Prison*, NACRO Briefing.

NACRO (1986) *News Digest* 37.

O'Donovan, K. (1984) 'The medicalisation of infanticide', *Criminal Law Review* 259–64.

O'Dwyer, J. and Carlen, P. (1985) 'Surviving Holloway and other women's prisons', in P. Carlen *et al. Criminal Women*, Cambridge: Polity Press.

O'Hagan, K. (1986) *Crisis Intervention in Social Services*, London: Macmillan.

Otto, S. (1981) 'Women, alcohol and social control', in B. Hutter and G. Williams (eds) *Controlling Women*, London: Croom Helm.

Pattullo, P. (1983) *Judging Women*, London: NCCL.

Pearson, R. (1976) 'Women defendants in magistrates' courts', *British Journal of Law and Society* 3: 265–73.

Peckham, A. (1985) *A Woman in Custody*, London: Fontana.

Phillipson, C. (1981) 'Women in later life', in B. Hutter and G. Williams (eds) *Controlling Women*, London: Croom Helm.

Plummer, K. (1979) 'Misunderstanding labelling perspectives', in D. Downes and P. Rock (eds) *Deviant Interpretations*, Oxford: Martin Robertson.

Pointing, J. (ed.) (1986) *Alternatives to Custody*, Oxford: Blackwell.

Pollak, O. (1950) *The Criminality of Women*, Philadelphia: University of Pennsylvania Press.

Powell, M. (1985) 'Court work', in H. Walker and B. Beaumont (eds) *Working with Offenders*, London: Macmillan.

Procek, E. (1980) *The Role of Psychiatry in the Social Control of Women*, University of Keele, unpublished PhD thesis.

Raynor P. (1978) 'Compulsory persuasion: a problem for correctional social work', *British Journal of Social Work* 8 (4): 411–24.

Raynor, P. (1985) *Social Work, Justice and Control*, Oxford: Blackwell.

Rock, P. (1973) *Deviant Behaviour*, London: Hutchinson.

Rose, N. (1987) 'Beyond the public/private division: law, power and the family', *Journal of Law and Society* 14 (1): 61–86.

Rutherford, A. (1986) *Growing Out of Crime*, Harmondsworth: Pelican.

Sebeok, T. (ed.) (1975) *The Tell-Tale Sign*, Peter de Ridder Press.

Smart, C. (1976) *Women, Crime and Criminology: A Feminist Critique*, London: Routledge & Kegan Paul.

Sudnow, D. (1965) 'Normal crimes: sociological features of the penal code', *Social Problems* 12: 255–70.

Szasz, T. (1973) *The Manufacture of Madness*, St Albans: Paladin.

Taylor, L. (1979) 'Vocabularies, rhetorics and grammar', in D.M. Downes and P. Rock (eds) *Deviant Interpretations*, Oxford: Martin Robertson.

Walker, H. (1985) 'Women's issues in probation practice', in H. Walker and B. Beaumont (eds) *Working with Offenders*, London: Macmillan.

Walker, H. and Beaumont, B. (1981) *Probation Work: Critical Theory and Socialist Practice*, Oxford: Blackwell.

Walker, H. and Beaumont, B. (eds) (1985) *Working with Offenders*, London: Macmillan.

Ward, E. (1985) *Father–Daughter Rape*, London: The Women's Press.

Willis, A. (1986) 'Help and control in probation: an empirical assessment of probation practice', in J. Pointing (ed.) *Alternatives to Custody*, Oxford: Blackwell.

Wilson, E. (1977) *Women and the Welfare State*, London: Tavistock.

Worrall, A. (1978) *A Double Exception: A Study of the Processing of Female Offenders in a Magistrates' Court*, unpublished MA dissertation, Centre for Criminology, University of Keele.

Worrall, A. (1981) 'Out of place: female offenders in court', *Probation Journal* 28 (3): 90–3.

Worrall, A. (1987a) *Nondescript Women? A Study of the Judicial Construction of Female Lawbreakers as Abnormal Criminals and Abnormal Women*, unpublished PhD thesis, available from University of Keele Library.

Worrall, A. (1987b) 'Sisters in law? Women defendants and women magistrates', in P. Carlen and A. Worrall (eds) *Gender, Crime and Justice*, Milton Keynes: Open University Press.

Worrall, A. (1989) 'Working with female offenders: beyond "Alternatives to Custody"?' *British Journal of Social Work* 19 (2): 77–93.

INDEX

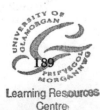

30 50 72 96